The Winning Weigh

Seven Steps to Healthier Living

Dr. Barry Simon
and
Dr. James Meschino

THE WINNING WEIGH:
SEVEN STEPS TO HEALTHIER LIVING

Copyright © 1993 by Simba Health Consultants Inc. and Meschino Nutritional Consultants. All rights reserved. No part of this book may be reproduced in any manner whatsoever without prior written permission from the publisher.

This book was developed and edited by Streit Bockus Publishing Services, Toronto
Editors: Dennis Bockus, Jennifer Dennison, Tanya Wood
Proofreaders: Dennis Bockus, Tanya Wood

Published and distributed by
Elite Publications Inc.
265 Rimrock Road, Unit 8
Downsview, Ontario
M3J 3C6

ISBN 0-9697011-0-1

Dedication

To our parents, for their love and support

My mother, Zel, taught me that dedication, commitment, and hard work are the only ways to achieve goals. My father, Morris, showed that love of learning and an easygoing nature could make the journey to the accomplishment of these goals fun and exciting. Together, by example, they have impressed upon me that compassion, learning from others, and giving are what life is all about.

Barry Simon

My mother, Lena, impressed upon me the virtues of patience, kindness, and compassion for others. She always encouraged me to follow my own path. My father, Armand, by his own example, taught me the importance of self-discipline, perseverance, and generosity toward others.

Jim Meschino

Acknowledgements

We would like to thank Fred Liberta for introducing us to each other. We are very grateful, Freddie. We wish to acknowledge Gordy Stefulic's encouragement and support during this project and Bob Sachter for his valued friendship and sound advice. We thank Ellen Feinman, Debra Korn, and Mindy Simon for their support and for their advice on ideas in the manuscript. We acknowledge the theoretical and clinical ideas of Dr. Aaron Beck (cognitive therapy), Dr. Roberto Assagioli (psychosynthesis), and Dr. Victor Frankl (logotherapy) who have provided inspiration and principles that have guided the development of steps 5 and 6. Many thanks are also due to Jennifer Dennison for her creativity and editing skills. and to Nadine Kostiuk, Alba Peddle, and Shelley Marple for their many hours of typing, formatting, and revision work. Special thanks to Dennis Bockus who did a wonderful job of editing the manuscript, but in addition provided guidance, support, and a belief in the worthiness of the project. Thanks also to Mark Klein and Michael Simon of Elite Publications who have given us the opportunity to potentially help more people in their journey toward healthier living.

Preface

If you read *The Winning Weigh,* it will teach you the basic nutritional knowledge you need to look after your body during your journey through life. It will tell you how to control your weight, restore your energy, and lower your risk of contracting diet-related illnesses. *The Winning Weigh* will also give you techniques to motivate you to actually use the knowledge you acquire.

Do not simply read this book. Reading is too passive unless it is accompanied by other action. To succeed with *The Winning Weigh,* you need to get involved in shaping your life. By interacting with the program, you will transform it into your own lifestyle story. You will see yourself beginning to change, physically as well as mentally, as you gradually adopt a healthier approach to living.

By reading and rereading this book, you will ultimately arrive at your own version of the Winning Weigh program. Become familiar with all the major sections of the book so that you can turn to them in those emergency moments. Carry the book with you as support during those overwhelming moments when old habits threaten to resurface.

The Winning Weigh will prepare you to deal with setbacks and savor your victories. Most important of all, it will help you live in the moment by being the best possible you!

Cautionary Note
The Winning Weigh provides a map for a lifetime journey toward healthier living. It does not provide therapeutic diets or nutritional therapies for particular ailments and is not intended to replace the advice of a personal physician or medical specialist. Since no program can consider all the health needs of every reader, we strongly recommend that you consult with your doctor before beginning to follow the *Winning Weigh's* nutritional, exercise, and psychological strategies for success. A complete examination is the first step in identifying your starting point, and it will help you modify the Winning Weigh program to suit your individual needs.

Many people have developed eating disorders over their lifetime. If you have suffered from anorexia or bulimia nervosa, you should not use this program without the guidance of a therapist or physician.

Physicians, dieticians, and any other health professionals who would like to know more about starting people on the Winning Weigh program should contact:

>The Winning Weigh
>c/o Dr. James Meschino
>Apex-Lawrence Medical Building
>960 Lawrence Ave. W., Suite 306
>Toronto, Ontario
>M6A 3B5

Questions specifically related to the psychology of wellness can be addressed to:

>Dr. Barry Simon
>36 Madison Avenue
>Toronto, Ontario
>M5R 2S1

In this book we have named some products solely for readers' information. None of these lists should be considered an endorsement of any given product. The information regarding the nutritional value of the various products was taken directly from their packages. This book is not meant to provide an exhaustive review of all the products available on the market.

Table of Contents

Foreword
Introduction 1

Step 1: Getting Started 7
Dieting: A Formula for Distress.................................7
    Diet Junkies...8
    Living in the Comfort Zone 9
    Your Mind/Body Rhythm 10
    Compassionate Commitment 12
    Lifestyle Script 12
Starting Right Now...15
Summary of Step 1..15
Looking Ahead 16

Step 2: Focusing on the Benefits................................17
    Physical Benefits...17
    Psychological Benefits 18
    The Successful Failure 19
Complex Carbohydrates 21
    Refined Sugars 24
    Complex Carbohydrate Energy 25
    Complex Carbohydrates and Athletic Performance........25
    Complex Carbohydrates and Weight Reduction 27
    Anti-Cancer Foods...29
        Protective Ingredient No. 1: Vitamin C 30
        Protective Ingredient No. 2: Vitamin E 31
        Protective Ingredient No. 3: Beta-Carotene 31
        Protective Ingredient No. 4: Indole Rings 31
        Protective Ingredient No. 5: Fiber......................32
    Starting Right Now...33
Fiber 35
    The Nature of Fiber 35
    Cholesterol Crunchers...36
    Colon Cleaners 39
        Foods High in Colon Cleaners............................41
    Fiber in Your Diet..41

- Starting Right Now... 42
- Fats 45
  - How Much Fat Is Enough? 45
  - The Dangers of Too Much Fat 46
    - Eating Fat Makes You Fat 48
  - Saturated Fat 48
  - Saturated Fat and Cholesterol 49
  - How Your Body Handles Cholesterol 51
    - The Big Plaque Attack 53
    - The Good Guys and the Bad Guys 54
    - Play It Smart, Play It Safe 55
  - Polyunsaturated Fats 56
    - An Extra Danger: Partially Hydrogenated Foods 57
  - Monounsaturated Fats 57
  - Omega 3 Fats 59
  - Fighting the Fat Temptation 60
  - Starting Right Now... 60
- Protein Foods and Their Nutrients 63
  - Protein from Low-Fat Dairy Foods 64
  - Calcium from Low-Fat Dairy Foods 65
  - Protein from Low-Fat Flesh Foods 67
  - Vitamin B_{12} 67
  - Iron 68
  - Protein in Complex Carbohydrates 69
  - Starting Right Now... 69
- Water and Other Fluids 71
  - Salt (Sodium) 72
    - The Dangers of a High-Sodium Diet 72
    - Cutting Back on Sodium 73
  - Sources of Fluids 76
    - Water 76
    - Coffee and Tea 77
    - Alcohol 77
    - Juice 78
  - Diet Soft Drinks and Soda Water 78
  - Starting Right Now... 78
- Exercise 79
  - The Importance of Aerobic Exercise 80

      Cardiovascular Benefits 80
      Stress Reduction 81
      Fat Reduction..82
      After the Exercise Stops 83
  The Benefits of Light Exercise...............................84
  Starting Right Now... 86

Step 3: Discovering the Formula 87
The Winning Weigh Program 87
  The Two Staples of the Winning Weigh Program............88
  The Winning Weigh Meal Plan 90
  The Vegetarian Option 92
  Other Elements of the Winning Weigh Program................92
      Oils 93
      Water 93
      Fiber 93
  Keeping on the Winning Weigh 94
  Starting Right Now... 95
Making the Program Work 97
  Using Substitutions to Make the Wish Come True 99
  The Emergency Snack 103
  A Typical Day with the Winning Weigh 104
  Starting Right Now... 105
Food Preparation Guide 107
  General Tips...107
  Low-Fat Flesh Protein Foods 107
  Low-Fat Dairy Protein......................................108
  Breakfast Cereals 109
  Bread 109
  Crackers and Biscuits 110
  Fruit..111
  Vegetables 111
  Grains...112
  Peas and Beans 112
  Pasta 113
  Oils 114
  Snack Foods and Desserts...............................114
  Beverages 115

- Dining at Restaurants 116
  - Chinese Restaurants 117
  - Italian Restaurants 117
  - Mexican Restaurants 118
  - Chicken Restaurants 118
  - Deli or Greasy Spoon Dining 118
  - Fast-Food Restaurants 119
- Combination Foods 119
- Recipes 121
- Your First Winning Weigh Shopping List.....................122
  - Beverages 122
  - Fruits and Vegetables 123
  - Bread Products 123
  - Cereals and Grains 124
  - Legumes 124
  - Low-Fat Flesh Proteins................................124
  - Low-Fat Dairy Protein 125
  - Miscellaneous 125
  - Occasional Foods 125
- Starting Right Now...126
- Future Trends: Designer Foods and Supplements...............127
- The Argument in Favor of Vitamin
  and Mineral Supplementation....................................128
- Sample Meals for Seven Days 137
  - Chicken Dishes...138
  - Fish Dishes and Seafood 138
  - Great Complex Carbohydrate Meals 139
  - Appetizers 140
  - Low-Fat Dairy Meals 140
  - Side Dishes...140
  - Homemade Desserts and Breads 140
- Seven Days on the Winning Weigh.............................141
  - Day One 141
  - Day Two 142
  - Day Three...143
  - Day Four 144
  - Day Five 145
  - Day Six 146

    Day Seven 147
    People Who Are Lactose- or Dairy Intolerant..............148
    Starting Right Now 149
Exercise 151
    The Light Activity Program: The Power Walker...........153
    The Wellness-Oriented Exerciser..................................154
        Types of Aerobic Exercise 157
    The Elite Athlete 158
    Long-Term Compliance..160
    Starting Right Now..163
    Summary 164
Looking Ahead...164

Step 4: Setting Your Goals..165
    How Motivated Are You? 165
    The Power of a Contract..174
    Time, Experience, and Repetition 175
    Personal Benefits 176
        External Benefits...176
        Internal Benefits 177
        Intangible Benefits..177
Starting Right Now...177
Summary for Step 4 178
Looking Ahead 178

Step 5: Jumping the Hurdles 179
Your Lifestyle Script 179
    Your Unconscious Mind 179
    Your Lifestyle Script...180
        Act I: The Blissful Binge...................................181
        Act II: The Perfect Forever Fantasy 183
        Act III: The Revolution......................................184
        The Never-Ending Cycle 185
        No Damage Done? Wrong!..............................188
    Your Role in Your Lifestyle Script.................................189
        Who Was That Last Night Anyway?................189
        Your Sedentary Slob...191
    Starting Right Now..192

Recognizing Your Sedentary Slob 193
   Sedentary Slob Activators 193
      Activator Category No. 1: Situations 194
      Activator Category No. 2: People 195
      Activator Category No. 3: Energy States 195
   Your Sedentary Slob Beliefs 196
   Your Thoughts: A Product of Beliefs 197
      1. Procrastinated Success 199
      2. Feeling Forecasting 199
      3. Disaster Thinking 200
      4. Blaming Others 202
      5. Blaming Yourself 202
      6. Weak and Dizzy 202
      7. Never, Ever Again 202
      8. And They Lived Happily Ever After 203
      9. Doing/Undoing 203
      10. Eureka 204
   Changing Your Thinking Style 204
   Starting Right Now... 205
Adopting a Winning Attitude 207
      Love 207
      Time 207
      Belief in Yourself 208
      Hard Work 208
   Breathing and Posturing: The Mind-Body Link 209
      Diaphragmatic Breathing 210
      Posturizing 211
   Visualizing a New You 211
      Relaxation 212
      Affirmations 214
   Your Wellness Image 214
   High-Risk Situations 218
   Starting Right Now... 219
Summary for Step 5 220

Step 6: Living in the Moment 223
      Playful and Powerful 223
What is "Living in the Moment"? 227

Intensity Levels 227
　　　　1. Overwhelming Intensity 228
　　　　2. Optimum Intensity 228
　　　　3. Insufficient Intensity 228
　　Your Internal Director..229
　　Making a 15-Minute Committnent 232
　　　　Action: Empowering Your Wellness Role..............232
　　Starting Right Now... 235
　Switching Out of Overwhelming Intensity 237
　　Seeing Your Way Out 242
　　Thinking Your Way Out 242
　　　　Rewriting The Script 243
　　　　The ABCs 248
　　Talking Your Way Out..249
　　　　Creating Your Sedentary Slob..................................249
　　　　Talking Your Way Out...250
　　　　Approach Number 1: Creating an Old Friend....252
　　　　Approach Number 2: Exaggerating the Outcome..252
　　　　Approach Number 3: Make My Day.................253
　　Acting Your Way Out...254
　　Starting Right Now...257
　Switching Out of Insufficient Intensity 259
　　Seeing Your Way Out 260
　　　　Health Visualization 260
　　　　Disease Visualization..261
　　Thinking Your Way Out 261
　　Acting Your Way Out 263
　　Your Wellness Journey 263
　　The Method in Five Scenes 265
　　Starting Right Now...270
　Summary for Step 6 271
　Looking Ahead... 271

Step 7: Becoming the Goal Today 273
　Staying on Track 273
　　The Three Daily Steps 275
　　　　Familiarize..275
　　　　Visualize..275
　　　　Diarize 276

The Evolution Process 277
　　　The Three Weekly Steps 277
　　　Bring in the Reinforcements 280
　　　　　　1. Health Magazines 280
　　　　　　2. Audio and Video Tapes 280
　　　　　　3. Pictures 281
　　　　　　4. Quotes 281
　　　　　　5. Getting Enough Rest 282
　　　　　　6. Positive People 282
　　　　　　7. The Winning Weigh 283
　　　Starting Right Now... 283
　　The Wellness Shift 285
　　　Starting Right Now... 288
　　Summary of Step 7 288
　　Appendix: The Winning Weigh Booster Plan 289

The Fiber Scoreboard 293

The Wellness Planner 305

The Daily Food, Fiber, and Activity Journal 323

The Weekly Body Shape Summary 326

INTRODUCTION

This book is for people who are overweight, out of shape, or feeling a lack of energy in their day-to-day lives. It is for people who realize that nutrition is important but who are confused by the vast amount of misinformation that has been passed along by pseudo-experts. It is for people who are alarmed by the staggering rates of heart disease, cancer, diabetes, and other degenerative disorders today. It is for people who already have started on the road to wellness and are looking for a sound nutrition program to complement their fitness routines and enhance their athletic performance. Finally, this book is for people who have never given much thought to nutrition.

Many people go through life not paying much attention to what they eat. Others wander from the latest diet book or program to the trendiest health club in search of the magic formula that will make them energetic and attractive for the rest of their lives. Many of these people are caught in what we call the Perfect Forever Fantasy. The Perfect Forever Fantasy is the hope that the latest magic formula will mark the start of a new and better life. Somehow all those established habits will be forgotten, and the new, healthy way of living will emerge effortlessly and last forever. Most weight-loss books cater to this fantasy. They provide regimented details, menus, and recipes. No thinking is required from the readers.

If you have tried these approaches, you probably know they don't work. The biggest problem in going on someone else's diet is that it is **someone else's diet.** This book helps you adopt habits that are appropriate to your personal tastes, timetables, and body rhythms.

Just as there is a law of gravity, there are natural laws of human behavior. Put simply, it is difficult to change behavior that has become established. The foods you like to eat and the activities and exercises you do become entrenched habits. We set out seven steps that you can follow to change your relationship with your health. Some diet books set out three or four of these steps, but they leave the process of change incomplete. Achieving long-term success is much easier for people who have the entire formula.

We wrote this book with one truth in mind: the small daily effort required to maintain the health of your physical body is not only worthwhile and within your ability, but it is the first essential step toward living a long, productive, and rewarding life. After all, your health is at the center of your existence.

As you assimilate our seven steps into your life one by one, you will eventually develop new wellness habits of eating and living. And these habits will transform you into a fitter, healthier, more energized, more shapely person — the person that nature intended you to be.

If you hear yourself saying, "Seven steps are too many!" or "There must be an easier way!" or "Nothing will happen to my health, so why bother!" you are in danger of wandering off once again in search of the unattainable. We have worked with enough people to know that the majority need all seven steps.

The Winning Weigh's seven-step formula is based on our knowledge that the energy and ingredients for success and health are not in a recipe or food calendar but in yourself. That's why you'll find **The Winning Weigh** has few actual recipes for meals. Instead, this book is the recipe for opening your life to health.

The first step in long-term success is focusing on the benefits. Before setting any goal, you want to know "What is in this for me?" When it comes to wellness, the benefit is simple — your health is the foundation for any of your life goals and dreams. No career, financial, spiritual, or family goal is unaffected by your health.

By picking up this book, you have already begun your process of change. The second step is to reconnect yourself to the natural laws of health. Living in our concrete, mechanical world, we often forget that we are part of nature. Nature is run by certain unalterable rules. Science has translated natural laws into lists of health-promoting and disease-promoting foods. We help you take the second step by defining for you the laws of nature as they apply to the foods you eat and the exercise you do. We help you separate scientific facts from unsubstantiated superstition.

Let's look at some of those facts. One out of every nine women in North America develops breast cancer. The statistics are basically the same for prostate cancer in men over the age of 60. One in twenty people will develop colon cancer, the second major cancer in North America. Approximately 50 percent of people die from heart and stroke problems, usually well before they have completed what should be their life expectancy. Beginning as early as 35 years of age for men and 45 years of age for women, the chances of an individual dying from coronary heart disease increases progressively and dramatically. Compared to other countries that routinely follow health-promoting dietary practices, our incidence of these diseases — along with diabetes, uterine cancer, and ovarian cancer — are absolutely frightening. The body of evidence makes one fact increasingly clear:

how you feed your body strongly determines your health potential and the likelihood that you will live longer.

To put it another way, there will probably be danger ahead of you if you do not act on the principles contained in ***The Winning Weigh.*** Right from the start, you must know that we are totally committed to helping you succeed in changing your disease-promoting patterns. As you discover the foods that increase your energy and protect your body against cancer and heart disease, you will find your commitment to wellness will grow. So Step 2 really reinforces Step 1 by giving you information about the benefits of a commitment to caring for your body.

You can be fit and healthy without becoming a health nut or a fitness fanatic. You don't have to grow bean sprouts or bake your own bread. ***The Winning Weigh*** shows you a balanced plan for wellness. It doesn't matter who you are; this book can help you succeed in using diet to create a healthier life for yourself.

After exploring the natural laws that affect health, Step 3 will show you a simple formula that will allow you to design healthy meals that suit your tastes and your life. Discovering how simple the Winning Weigh formula is should encourage you to actively promote your health each time you open the refrigerator or enter a restaurant. Our formula, which we call the two-staple system, provides the correct balance of nutrients to follow your genetic blueprints for optimal health and disease prevention.

Learning the formula is not enough. You need to strengthen your commitment so that you don't wander away from the program during parties and business lunches or at the end of a long day. We quickly realized what any successful person knows intuitively — you don't reach a long-term goal unless you have specifically defined what the goal is. Step 4 will help you establish your goals. The very step of writing down your goal will help you mobilize your energy to achieve your specific objective.

We could have stopped the book with Step 4 if human beings didn't have habits. Your favorite foods are old friends you turn to during lonely, sad, frustrating, or tired times. These relationships with food create and entrench automatic patterns of behavior. Step 5 focuses on overcoming your habits. We call it "Jumping the Hurdles." We help you discover your personal attitude toward food and exercise. You may discover your own version of a Sedentary Slob within you. That's the part of you that believes fatty foods are fantastic and exercise is something you do when the channel changer is broken on your TV set. We will delve into your unconscious using simple word games and you will begin to unravel the subconscious hold your Sedentary Slob has on you.

If you have ever tried even one wellness or diet program, you know how high-fat, high-calorie foods begin to cry out "Eat me" the very minute after you swear to never eat them again. Step 5 helps you through the difficult period of battling your unconscious to change your eating habits.

The last two steps evolved over years of working with people. We give you a series of techniques to help you overcome the urge to eat late at night, at weddings, or any other times you start to feel your old way taking over. These exercises are the fire extinguishers that will put out your temptations to abandon wellness. We end the book and send you on your way with some tips on how to stay on track.

The heart of success is enthusiasm. Enthusiasm is the energy that powers all major achievements in life. Our experiences have shown that a person must be motivated and possessed by the desire to succeed. Many programs fall short. They provide the nutritional guidelines but fail to prescribe a proven method to put that knowledge into action. ***The Winning Weigh*** will kindle your enthusiasm by teaching you the skills of goal-setting, psychological energizing, changing your self-image, breaking old habits, and enjoying a new you. We have taken principles that are applied daily in successful businesses, psychotherapy sessions, and motivational programs and reoriented them into advice for you on how to set health goals and succeed in accomplishing the goals you set. Gradually, the Winning Weigh principles will become a natural extension of your life, a part of who you are.

Good health does not just come from following a set of rules; it is an attitude. You can achieve your wellness goals. We will help you, as we've helped others, to overcome your self-limiting, negative beliefs and past failures and to be reborn to good health. You are about to experience a breakthrough by discovering the joys and benefits of the Winning Weigh lifestyle. So get ready, and let's move the action forward.

STEP 1   GETTING STARTED

Dieting: A Formula for Distress

Don't think of your diet as just some two-week guide to losing ten pounds. Your diet is your long-term attitude to food. The word comes from the Greek word meaning "a way of life," and you will be healthier if you think of it that way.

Whether you are a sleek long-distance runner, an aerobic enthusiast, a trim couch potato, or 25 pounds overweight, your diet has a lot to do with the way you live and how long you live. Your diet could lead you to obesity, clogged coronary arteries, or cancer. Your personal way of living is either your own formula for distress or health.

We certainly live in a strange society. We take great pride in our freedom of choice, yet we all tend to chase the same goals. Nowhere is this external standard of success more evident than in the area of health and beauty. We measure ourselves by the same standards we apply to movie stars, fashion models, and athletes to determine whether we are acceptable. Advertising campaigns convince us to select food based on image and taste rather than nutrition.

Many people react to this external control in one of two ways. Some become diet junkies, chronically trying and failing at new weight-loss or health programs. They read the checkout-counter tabloids to discover which movie star is endorsing the latest diet plan promising that they can drop ten pounds over a long weekend. Unfortunately, all they lose is three days. In disgust, they swear off dieting until the next foolproof program comes along.

Other people react by living in the comfort zone, eating whatever they want regardless of the health consequences. Food doesn't cause them emotional stress. They are manipulated into following a health-damaging lifestyle by clever advertising campaigns, restaurant-size helpings, and fast-food recipes. They may have some nutritionally sound eating habits, but they have not made any strong commitment to healthy living. Eventually, most of these people become obese or develop serious health problems.

The long-term health decisions of both these groups are determined by outside forces. In both cases, diet is a formula for distress. ***The Winning Weigh is designed to help you regain control over health decisions.***

Diet Junkies

Many people spend most of their lives trying to lose 25 to 30 pounds as quickly as possible. Unfortunately, they use diet programs that have all the ingredients needed to guarantee failure. ***Evidence shows that 95 percent of dieters eventually regain all the weight they lose.*** You have to wonder whether the designers of diet programs know exactly what they are doing – creating a 95 percent return rate among their clients. The diet industry generates a billion dollars a year because it fails most of its customers.

If you have trouble accepting this contention, just look at how the diet process works. Most dieters feel helpless and out of control; they are desperately searching for a magical cure that requires little effort. Along comes a program that promises just that. Dutifully, they swear off "bad" foods (however bad is defined by the particular program). The strict regimen they adopt makes them long for treats and despise "good foods" for being boring; nonetheless, they follow to the word every direction their dietary guide dictates to them. Eventually, however, in a moment of "weakness," they find themselves back in their old patterns – demoralized and feeling even worse about themselves. They blame themselves for failure instead of recognizing the weaknesses inherent in the program.

Not surprisingly, these dieters begin, once again, to look for another outside solution. They don't realize that the problem lies in the diets themselves – they just don't work.

Unfortunately, dieters are typically very critical of themselves, always focusing on their inadequacies. Their feelings about themselves are determined by the reactions of others. They long to get recognition from the outside world in order to feel better about themselves, but even their successes can't provide the recognition and admiration they hope to get because they demand so much. They become like sheep, passively following the herd up ahead. This loss of control increases the weight-loss dieters' feelings of distress. Eventually, they move on to a new program, hoping to improve the way other people see them, hoping to live up to the standards of others. Sadly, these programs were not designed to help them in the first place.

Living in the Comfort Zone

Many North Americans don't understand the emotional battles of the long-term dieter. They live in a comfort zone, eating whatever is most convenient and pleasurable with little regard for their health. Eventually, following this pattern may lead them to become overweight or develop mild diabetes. Instead of becoming depressed or anxious about what they are doing to themselves, they simply go on eating whatever they want, failing to appreciate the grave impact that their poor dietary habits can have on their well-being. Living in their comfort zone merely delays the emotional distress they will ultimately encounter.

Or course, not everyone is this extreme. Many people apply some nutritional knowledge to their eating habits in a random sort of way. One person might avoid all dairy products but eat red meat. Another will avoid beef but be unable to resist chocolate. Still other people recognize the connection between fat and heart disease, know about the dangers of too much cholesterol, and recognize the value of vegetables, yet still find it hard to make health-promoting decisions consistently. They have the facts but lack the formula to make lasting changes.

Instead of making conscious choices, people in the comfort zone react to the millions of advertising dollars spent to convince them how pleasurable high-fat foods are. Have you ever seen a commercial show a fat, lonely man eating in a fast-food restaurant? Of course not – it's always a thin, beautiful family, sharing a loving moment. Who wouldn't want to be part of that image and feeling? And yes, it does affect you. Do you really think advertisers would spend their money if it didn't?

Your Mind/Body Rhythm

With all these external forces influencing your wellness choices, you need a way of evaluating what is right for you. That standard should be set by your own mind/body rhythm. Your mind/body rhythm is a realistic balance between your desires and the actual requirements of your body.

Unfortunately, your body is the silent partner in this formulation. Certainly, it gives some clues when it isn't functioning properly, but for the most part, it quietly adapts to the treatment you give it. If you eat foods that are high in fat or cholesterol, it doesn't call out to you, "Hey! We're putting on weight around the hips!" or "Your coronary arteries are filling up with fatty plaque." It just silently accumulates layer upon layer of excess fat. However, if you exercise regularly, your heart gets stronger and pumps more blood with each contraction. If you eat high-fiber, low-fat foods, your cholesterol count comes down and your arteries clear. This a partnership: your body will react to **your** decisions; it will change, adapt, and be responsive to your conscious choices. You just need to recognize good choices and to make them consistently.

Until now, you may have been guided by diet programs and advertising campaigns. For long-term success, however, you need to realize how your body silently adapts in the short term. By focusing your mind and your attention on the way your body changes, on your ***mind/body rhythm,*** you can reach your long-term wellness goals. You need to begin to listen for this rhythm, to identify and develop it over the weeks and months. Your only indicator of success should be what your body is telling you.

On the Winning Weigh program, you should not feel as if you're on a diet, at least in the way you are used to thinking about diets. The Winning Weigh is a way of life that you tailor to your own emotional and physical needs. No two bodies have exactly the same shape, height, metabolism, or athletic potential. Each body has its own strengths and weaknesses. You need to realize the implications of this fact. Are you judging your success or failure against external standards? Instead of seeing your strengths, are you focusing on your "defects"? Do you feel that you're not tall enough, slim enough, fast enough, or sexy enough? Enough for what? To measure up to movie stars, aerobic teachers, models, athletes, or even your next-door neighbor? If you answered "yes" to these questions, you need to adjust your expectations to the real you. You need to get in touch with your own mind/body rhythm instead of trying to adopt someone else's life.

If you are a diet junkie, the typical diet program sets up reinforcement for the attitude that you're not good enough. If you live in the comfort zone, you undervalue your potential by not demanding enough of yourself. In both cases, you need to set specific, personal, realistic goals. Look at your own potential as the gauge of what you can achieve. Then you will begin to be the best possible you.

Here's an example. Your ideal body weight might be ten pounds above average for your height. It is only common sense that some people will be above the average and some will be below it. You may think you will feel better if you lose ten pounds. But if you do it by starving yourself and immediately gain it back again, then you will only succeed in demoralizing and frustrating yourself. You should look beyond weight and measurements to factors such as your fat intake, the amount of fiber you eat, and your physical fitness. Our patients always tell us that they knew intuitively that typical diets wouldn't be effective or that high-fat food couldn't be good for them. In contrast, when we teach them the Winning Weigh formula for recapturing their lost mind/body rhythm, the program feels right to them.

Compassionate Commitment

To succeed in the long run, you need what we call ***compassionate commitment.*** This state requires that you understand and accept yourself as you are while learning to stick to realistic goals that will make you as healthy as possible.

Compassionate commitment is a very difficult concept to adopt, both for people in the comfort zone and for diet junkies. If you are a diet junky, you will have no difficulty committing yourself to restrictive programs, but you may find it very hard to develop compassion for yourself and for your own unique mind/body rhythm. Don't be afraid to settle for a weight that is higher than what you had hoped for. Deep down you probably know that the typical weight-loss diet will fail you. Learn to have compassion for the pain and struggle you have already been through and begin to discover who ***you*** are.

People living in the comfort zone have a great deal of compassion for their desires but little compassion for or commitment to their bodies. If you fit into this group, you'll need to re-evaluate your commitment. Begin by asking yourself how many of your long-term goals you can enjoy if you are seriously ill. What about your family? Travel? Retirement? Probably all of these would be affected by the results of years of undisciplined eating.

Lifestyle Script

The Winning Weigh is about changing you from the ***inside out.*** We have found that simply setting your new goals and adopting a compassionate commitment to your mind/body rhythm is not enough for long-term success. That's because of your subconscious lifestyle script. Your lifestyle script is based on a lifetime of experiences and beliefs about yourself, about food, and about exercise. It is the unconscious story that guides your behavior. A chronic overeater might follow an automatic script of overeating, then attempting a restrictive diet, and eventually rebelling against the tyrannical program to return to self-indulgence. Ideas like "chocolate is fun" and "salad is boring" reflect this automatic script. Chocolate and salad aren't inherently fun or boring; it's your attitude that endows foods with particular attributes.

People in the comfort zone also follow a lifestyle script that ignores the facts. Anyone who thinks that high-fat foods are fun is ignoring the obvious fact that nothing is enjoyable about heart disease or strokes. You need to see clearly how your habits put your health at risk. Once you discover your blind spots, you can start finding solutions. You can ask:

> What eating and exercise habits are in the best interests of my body?
> What are my personal risk factors and how can I protect myself?
> What is my ideal body weight, as opposed to the average given on the insurance tables?
> How can I develop a wellness program that is in harmony with my lifestyle?
> How important is my health to me?

In time, you will see life as a series of choices about health instead of a battle between boring foods and fun foods. You won't look at a bowl of ice cream and label it as good or bad; instead, you will assess whether eating it is in your best interest. If that sounds boring, then you are just the person who needs this book. ***The Winning Weigh*** will help rekindle your lost love affair with your health.

You might ask, "When will this rebirth begin?" Well, it begins this very moment. Life is a series of moments and in any one of them you can choose to make new commitments and choices. Most health programs last only for a specific length of time or focus exclusively on the long-term perspective. ***The Winning Weigh*** highlights ***this moment.*** Ultimately, regardless of present worries or past regrets, the only real commitment you can make is in *this* moment. You can hope to be different, but the present moment is the only time you can *become* different. All of your long-term choices are based upon what you do on a day-to-day, moment-by-moment basis. That is why we spend a lot of time teaching you how to focus on this moment – to see your unconscious script, to recognize your possibilities, and to use our techniques to make a conscious choice.

The concept of living in the moment stresses that a plan is only real if you actualize it in your daily life. You have to use a plan, not just think about it. Even while reading this book, you will find your motivation increasing and decreasing. Make notes in the margins of facts, ideas, and images that increase your enthusiasm. We will show you how to focus this enthusiasm into a force that will guide your behavior.

You could think of **The Winning Weigh** as your guide on a wellness climb up a high mountain. Standing at the base of the mountain, you are unsure how high you will go or what route you will take. We will direct, teach, and excite you into the wellness shift, but ultimately you will need to journey off on your own. We will show you how to get back on track if you wander off, but it's up to you to stay on your own path.

One warning before you begin. The road to wellness passes through times of crisis and fear. In fact, these feelings show that you are on the right track. The Japanese word for "crisis" has two symbols. The first stands for danger, while the second stands for opportunity. Any time you attempt to change your unconscious mind and behave in a new way, you will feel the danger as well as the opportunity. If you follow the Winning Way, we hope to help you get through the danger and nurture the opportunity to create a new you.

So begin your wellness journey with the attitude that you will be the best possible you. You probably won't be a famous model or a star athlete, but you'll quickly realize that having a fit, healthy body is within your power. We have yet to meet anyone who wasn't happier with themselves after mastering these skills. From this point forward, it's all up to you.

Starting Right Now . . .

In the Wellness Planner (p. 305), fill out the chart "My Wellness Starting Point." As you follow the Winning Weigh program, you can flip back and see how much your wellness has improved.

Summary of Step 1

1. Everyone has a relationship to food that is called their diet. Most people use unrealistic ideals, such as fashion models, movie stars, or sports heroes to set their own health and wellness standards.

2. Diet junkies continually join the latest weight-loss program to overcome feelings of helplessness about being unable to achieve their ideal external standards.

3. People who live in their comfort zone indulge in the fast-food fantasy land created by clever advertising agencies. Food is purely a desire. There is no regard for its relationship to the risk of heart disease, cancer, and other disorders.

4. Your mind/body rhythm is the balance between your desires and the needs and requirements of your body.

5. Long-term change demands that you slowly transform how you feel about yourself and your body.

6. To arrive at your lifestyle goals you will need to have compassionate commitment to your ability to change, while respecting who you are at this very moment. This compassionate commitment to long-term change is the basis of the Winning Weigh program.

Looking Ahead . . .

The next step will build a foundation of well-being that will empower you to make health-promoting choices. By being aware of the basic facts about carbohydrates, fiber, fat, protein, water, and exercise, you will see the concrete benefits of making the wellness shift.

STEP 2   FOCUSING ON THE BENEFITS

Good dietary habits can significantly improve your chances of living a long, healthy, and productive life. You may want to lose a few pounds, and that's great, but the Winning Weigh program is intended to provide more than a short-term fix. Rather, it will help you develop a new relationship with your body and empower you to make wellness choices consistently.

Making these big changes is actually just a small task. Usually, they only require adjusting a few things in your lifestyle. Yet we know from experience with the people we have counselled over the years that *the more real to you the benefits of the Winning Weigh program are, the better your chances for long-term success.* So in order to improve your chances of success, you must take the second step up the wellness ladder – you must focus on the benefits of the Winning Weigh program, both physical and psychological.

Physical Benefits

In our society, 50 percent of all deaths are caused by cardiovascular disease and another 20 percent by cancer. Most of these lives could have been extended through proper eating and exercise habits. The Winning Weigh program is designed to keep your blood cholesterol count and blood pressure down and to keep your resistance to cancer and other degenerative diseases up. In fact, many of our patients have reduced their cholesterol counts enough to cut their risk of heart disease in half. Cancers of the colon, rectum, breast, ovaries, prostate, and cervix are especially responsive to wellness habits. *Gori and Wynder, two prominent cancer researchers, have estimated that 60 percent of all cancers in women and 40 percent of all cancers in men are directly related to faulty dietary patterns.*

The Winning Weigh program can also help you attain your ideal body weight. Not only will this accomplishment make you look and feel better, but it will decrease your risk of heart disease, adult-onset diabetes, gall bladder disease, degenerative arthritis, and high blood pressure. Indeed, the simple process of shedding some excess weight is in itself a first step on the road to wellness for many people. Being at or near your ideal weight is a protective measure against heart disease, cancer, and other health problems.

Finally, the Winning Weigh program will boost your level of energy. Increased energy will improve your performance at work and at leisure. Because you'll feel better physically and have more energy, you'll be able to do more and be more productive. Many of our patients tell us that they feel physically rejuvenated, with more energy than they've had for years.

Psychological Benefits

The psychological benefits you can achieve on the Winning Weigh program are just as important as the physical benefits. Knowing that you are making headway with a goal is an important benefit in itself. As you follow the Winning Weigh program, you may watch your weight go down, your energy level go up, or your time for a five-mile run improve. As you begin to benefit from the program, you will realize that you are making headway with your life. This realization, in turn, leads to a greater sense of self-esteem. Feeling better about yourself will make you more successful in all aspects of your life.

You should realize that your wellness progress will directly influence your work life, your social life, and your sex life. People who report to us on the inner sense of accomplishment that comes from meeting their goals often talk about how they feel a greater sense of power and confidence in all areas of their lives.

You might experience better mental clarity. Your exercise

routine will have a calming effect on the day-to-day stresses of life. Being healthier means you will look better, which can be an important factor in preserving a healthy self-image. With increased vitality, you will find greater richness in your life. The intangible benefit of being happy with yourself as you move closer to achieving your wellness goals may be the most important benefit of all.

The Successful Failure

Unfortunately, in today's world our lives are frequently out of balance. Many people push themselves to the limit, sacrificing their health in their quest for financial success. They get too little sleep, eat high-fat foods, and avoid physical activity. This lifestyle is out of balance with the genetic blueprints for good health. It accelerates the process of degenerative change in your body. Health is at the center of your existence. All other dimensions of your life will be severely impaired if you develop cancer or heart disease. Being healthy allows you to achieve your potential in all other aspects of your life.

To fully realize all the benefits that being healthy will provide for you, you must first understand the impact that your choices of food and activity have on your well-being. In this step, Focusing on the Benefits, you will learn how various foods and physical activity affect your metabolism and your health. Complex carbohydrates, proteins, fats, fiber, water, nutrients, and exercise all interact to promote health or to promote disease. Once you have the facts, you can decide. You will be able to envision how each food you eat will either enhance or disrupt your body's ability to function. The power will be in your hands.

As you gain this knowledge, identify the benefits that mean the most to you. Remember: *the more real to you the benefits of the Winning Weigh program are, the better your chances for long-term success.* Decide which benefits are of greatest importance to you and then zero in on these factors as a way of helping you remain committed to the program. Whenever you must make a choice affecting your health, ask yourself: "Is this in line with the health benefits that I want to achieve?" If you truly want to change your habits, you must remain in touch with the benefits of making consistent wellness choices.

Rather than thinking of foods as "good" or "bad," you will learn how different foods affect your body and how to recognize those that will contribute to your health. You can then rely upon that knowledge to help you make a choice in the moment. By using this information in a consistent, practical way, you will soon reap the benefits of wellness in your daily life.

Complex Carbohydrates

To develop a fit, trim, healthy body, eat complex carbohydrate foods. These foods come from the land – fruits, vegetables, grains (rice, corn, oats, barley, etc.), cereal products (bread, high-fiber breakfast cereals, pasta, etc.), and legumes (beans and peas).

Your body uses complex carbohydrate foods as the principal source of fuel to power your organs, tissues, and cells. Complex carbohydrates are a high-octane energy source. In fact, the natural laws that govern human health dictate that 55 to 65 percent of all the calories you consume each day should come from complex carbohydrate foods.

There are good reasons for putting complex carbohydrate foods at the centre of your diet. Complex carbohydrate foods contain vitamin C and beta-carotene, two of the most powerful cancer-fighting nutrients. Other complex carbohydrate foods provide dietary fiber, which can reduce the risk of colon cancer, improve the elimination of wastes, and lower cholesterol levels, thus reducing the chance of a heart attack or stroke. In short, complex carbohydrate foods boost your energy, reduce your risk of cancer, help keep your cholesterol in check, enhance your athletic performance, and enable your body to burn excess fat so that you maintain your ideal weight.

Typically, North Americans eat only half the amount of complex carbohydrates that their bodies need each day. This serious transgression against the natural laws of health contributes to the premature development of heart disease, strokes, and many cancers and to the overwhelming number of people in our society who are overweight. If you can make complex carbohydrates constitute 55 to 65 percent of your daily calories, you will have started toward a healthier life.

Now don't panic! We are not talking about a nutrition program that forces you to grow your own alfalfa sprouts and subsist on nothing but rabbit food for the rest of your life. Your body is more accommodating than that, and we aren't intending to make your life that uninteresting. There is such a wide variety of complex carbohydrates available that making them your predominant dietary staple will be easy once you get the hang of it.

Some complex carbohydrates are foods that you would probably list immediately as staples in a healthy diet. Look at the following list:

1. fresh fruit, such as apples, pears, plums, strawberries, papayas, mangoes, melons, oranges, and grapefruit
2. salad vegetables, such as lettuce, tomatoes, and cucumbers
3. starchy vegetables, such as potatoes and squash
4. cruciferous vegetables, including Brussels sprouts, broccoli, cauliflower, and cabbage
5. peas, both fresh and dried
6. beans, both fresh and dried, especially kidney beans and chick-peas
7. grains, including rice, oats, corn, barley, buckwheat, oatmeal, and bulgur wheat

In addition to the naturally occurring complex carbohydrates listed above, there are complex carbohydrates that have been modified for preservation and storage. For the most part, these are foods that you purchase in a can (for instance, chick-peas or tomato sauce), a bottle (orange juice), a jar (fruit jam), a bag (spaghetti noodles or bread), or a box (high-fiber cereal).

Each of the modified complex carbohydrates listed in Exhibit 2–1 behaves like a naturally-occurring complex carbohydrate once it is in your body. This makes these modified products perfectly acceptable foods to use as complex carbohydrate staples.

Not all natural foods should be part of your healthy diet. Nuts, seeds (pumpkin seeds, sunflower seeds, etc.), olives, and avocadoes have a fat content too high for us to consider them to be good staple foods. In later chapters, we will discuss the health benefits of using peanut oil and olive oil in preparing meals, but start with the general rule that eating nuts (with the exception of chestnuts), olives, or any seeds is a departure from your new

Exhibit 2–1
Modified Complex Carbohydrates

1. Fruit
   - frozen, with no added sugar
   - dried, with no added sugar
   - canned, in its own juice, with no added sugar
   - juices (1/4 glass of juice with 3/4 glass of water is the best ratio)
   - whole-fruit jams that are high in fiber and low in white sugar

2. Cereal products
   - high-fiber breakfast cereals
   - pasta and other noodles
   - bread, bagels, and low-fat biscuits
   - pizza dough

3. Clear broth soups
   - chicken noodle
   - minestrone
   - barley

Winning Weigh lifestyle. They add too many calories of fat to your diet, and too much fat of any kind speeds up degenerative processes in your body. Eating some avocado occasionally is not going to destroy your health, but those occasions should be very infrequent.

The distinguishing feature of complex carbohydrates foods lies in the way your body digests them and uses them for energy. As their name implies, complex carbohydrate foods have a somewhat complicated structural arrangement; consequently, it takes your digestive enzymes a fair bit of time to unravel these foods and release the individual carbohydrate sugars. Once released, these carbohydrate sugars pass into the bloodstream where they will ultimately become blood sugar, or glucose. The cells pick up the sugar from the bloodstream and use it as a source of energy. It doesn't matter if you eat a potato, a bowl of rice, a plate of pasta, a slice of bread, a piece of fruit, or a salad, the carbohydrate sugars in these foods will be slowly released by your digestive enzymes allowing a steady but controlled rise in blood sugar levels. Some of the blood sugar is used immediately and some is stored in the liver. Between meals, the liver releases these stored sugars to the bloodstream to match the energy needs of the body.

Many people fail to consume adequate amounts of complex carbohydrate foods, so their blood sugar often falls to low levels two or three hours after a meal. This condition is known as *hypoglycemia,* which literally means "low blood sugar". The symptoms of hypoglycemia include fatigue, an inability to concentrate, lethargy, irritability, nervousness, confusion, dull headaches, escalating hunger, and cravings for something sweet. Hypoglycemia affects the brain and nervous system most dramatically, because these nerve tissues rely on blood sugar for the energy to perform their functions.

So, failing to eat enough complex carbohydrate foods can bring on hypoglycemic symptoms between meals. In turn, this condition triggers the craving for something sweet. You may devour a couple of donuts or a chocolate bar to restore blood glucose levels quickly. These sweets contain refined carbohydrates, especially white sugar, which do tremendous damage to your body in the long run. Coffee with added sugar is especially potent. The caffeine in the coffee stimulates your liver to release whatever carbohydrate sugar it has available, and the added white sugar in the coffee doubles the fix.

Refined Sugars

Sugars may be consumed as white sugar, brown sugar, honey, or syrup. Unlike the complex carbohydrates, refined sugars are very easy for the digestive system to break down and absorb. They are absorbed into the bloodstream extremely quickly, resulting in a rapid elevation of blood sugar levels. The pancreas must then respond by pumping large quantities of insulin to the bloodstream to bring the level of blood sugar down to normal. Over your lifetime, the daily intake of refined sugars can oversensitize the pancreas so that it secretes more and more insulin. The insulin pushes blood sugar levels down, recreating the craving for sweets.

This repeating cycle is a common nutritional imbalance in our society. You can see its results in the number of overweight people. In response to the refined sugar bombardment, the liver begins to convert some extra carbohydrate sugars into fat. Weight gain is not the only problem resulting from this process. Some of the fat is stored and some circulates in the bloodstream as triglycerides. Elevated levels of triglycerides are a major contributing factor to heart attacks and strokes. The sugar fix cycle can kill you.

Complex Carbohydrate Energy

One of the most common complaints heard in doctors' offices is that people feel tired all the time. "Doctor, I feel so tired. Is there anything I can do about it?" When you consider that most people are walking around with their carbohydrate fuel tank less than half full at the best of times, it's no wonder that they are so tired.

Complex carbohydrates store the energy that plants originally trapped from sunlight in their chemical structure. When your body burns carbohydrate sugar, that energy is released to your tissues to power the vital processes of life. Your body's engine runs best on complex carbohydrate fuel. It burns cleanly, leaving no toxic residue to clog up your metabolic machinery. It is truly the high-octane energy source of the human body.

Complex Carbohydrates and Athletic Performance

Eating enough complex carbohydrate foods is also important for enhancing athletic performance. Your muscles can absorb and store carbohydrate sugars. These carbohydrates provide some of the energy for physical activity. Regularly exercised muscles can store double the amount of carbohydrate sugar, giving you more strength and endurance.

When a muscle has depleted its reserve of carbohydrate sugars during exercise, it becomes fatigued and soon reaches the point of complete exhaustion. During exercise that requires prolonged endurance (jogging, cycling, swimming), muscles extract carbohydrate sugars from the bloodstream at a rate 30 to 40 times faster than during rest or light activity. Those sugars are drawn from the liver.

A diet rich in complex carbohydrates keeps the supply of carbohydrate sugar stored in your liver and muscles high. This supply helps prevent your blood sugar levels from falling during exercise.

In marathon running, an empty carbohydrate fuel tank is known as "hitting the wall." Sometimes, at around the 20-mile mark of a 26.2-mile (42 km) marathon, the runners may begin to slow down, becoming weak and dizzy. Often, they can only walk the last few miles, if they can continue at all. What has happened is that the muscles have exhausted their stores of carbohydrates, and the liver can no longer maintain normal blood sugar levels. The brain and nervous system, deprived of the energy that they need to function properly, may cause so much dizziness that the runner falls. Athletes in many sports can suffer from carbohydrate depletion.

Athletes refer to the intake of a diet rich in complex carbohydrate foods as carb loading. By getting regular exercise and following the Winning Weigh program, you can expand your liver and muscle carbohydrate stores daily to provide you with a winning edge in your athletic pursuits. Carb loading will enhance both your endurance fitness level and your muscular strength.

Complex Carbohydrates and Weight Reduction

It's frightening how many people we meet are afraid to eat bread, pasta, or potatoes because they think those foods will make them fat. To us, this belief proves that many people are confused about how their bodies use the foods they eat. Don't avoid complex carbohydrate foods. Instead, start concentrating on them as a way to get back to an ideal weight and maintain it for a lifetime. It can be easy. Most of the people we have on the Winning Weigh program tell us, "I'm losing weight, and I don't even feel as if I'm dieting." They are really saying that they are not bothered by the unpleasant side effects associated with most diets: hunger, headaches, and irritability. Because many of the unpleasant aspects of diets are gone, the Winning Weigh approach has a much better chance of succeeding than fad diets do.

There are five important ways that complex carbohydrate foods help your body naturally attain and maintain your ideal weight:

1. Complex carbohydrates have less than half as many calories as the same amount of fat. One gram of a complex carbohydrate has four calories; one gram of fat has nine calories.
2. Studies have repeatedly demonstrated that our bodies do not absorb 10 to 20 percent of the calories in many complex carbohydrate foods. This fact is especially true for starchy foods, such as pasta, bread, legumes, and rice. Ironically, these are the very foods that many overweight people avoid. Our digestive enzymes cannot finish the job of breaking down these starchy complex carbohydrates foods in the small intestines. Partially digested food passes into the large intestine where no further absorption can take place. In a sense, these are free calories! Next time you look at a calorie counter, you can subtract 10 to

20 percent of the calories listed for starchy complex carbohydrates foods.
3. Complex carbohydrate foods require a lot of energy to digest. These energy calories are given off as heat from your body instead of being stored as fat. This process is called ***thermogenesis,*** which literally means "heat-producing."

   When your diet is high in complex carbohydrate foods, you burn more calories as heat after a meal. If you eat more complex carbohydrates than your liver can store, 23 percent of the extra calories are given off as heat from your body and the rest is converted into fat. In contrast, when you eat fat, it is digested, absorbed, assimilated, transported, and stored as fat with an efficiency rate of 93 percent. (These percentages were derived from a 1987 article by W.P.T. James, published in the American Journal of Clinical Nutrition.) Overeating carbohydrate foods, even refined sugars, is much less damaging to you than eating fat.
4. Starchy complex carbohydrate foods such as bread, pasta, rice, and bananas make you feel full after a meal. They actually shut off the hunger message from your brain. Nutritionists call this feeling ***satiety.*** Eliminating that feeling of hunger is a integral part of weight loss. Diets that require people to go around feeling hungry all the time are certain to fail. Fatty foods also produce that feeling of satiety, but they are much higher in calories, as well as being more damaging to your health in other ways. When you eat fat, you get fat. We'll be looking at fats in an upcoming section.
5. Complex carbohydrate foods provide the chemical links necessary to burn off body fat. In fact, if your carbohydrate intake is too low, you cannot completely break down your body fat. This inability makes it difficult for you to shed extra pounds. It also means that you build up toxic wastes (***ketone bodies***) in your system, causing headaches, dehydration, and overwhelming hunger pangs.

It's ironic that so many people stop eating bread, pasta, rice, peas, beans, and potatoes in their attempts to lose weight. They should take the opposite approach. No wonder 95 percent of all dieters regain the weight they lose; they're working against their bodies' metabolisms and setting the stage for long-term failure. It's not the bread and pasta you eat that makes you fat; it's the high-fat butter and sauces you put on them that do the damage. How many overweight vegetarians have you met? By themselves, starchy complex carbohydrates are tailor-made diet foods. So, when we present you with the Winning Weigh nutrition program, you will find a predominance of carbohydrate foods.

Anti-Cancer Foods

The value of complex carbohydrates goes beyond boosting your energy level and keeping you trim. A large number of complex carbohydrate foods also contain nutrients that substantially reduce your risk of developing many forms of cancer. These nutrients are discussed below and summarized in Exhibit 2–2.

Medical researchers refer to cancer-causing agents as free radicals. This term can be used to describe any compound that is chemically unstable and thus very reactive. As a rule, free radicals do their damage by aggressively attacking the genetic material of the cells they come in contact with, altering their genetic codes.

You have probably heard warnings from environmentalists about the dangers from free radicals that arise from food processing, soil treatment, and air pollution. The benzopyrene and ozone found in automobile emissions are particularly potent sources of free radicals. You should also be concerned about the use of nitrates as fertilizers and preservatives, since these nitrates can form nitrosamines, which are powerful carcinogens in humans.

It may surprise you to learn that some of the oxygen that you breathe gets transformed into oxygen radicals during the course of normal metabolism. These oxygen radicals cause damage to body cells and tissues. If you have ever cut open an apple and left it exposed to the air for a few minutes, you know that the exposed surface turns brown. This change in color is caused by oxygen radical attack. The same kind of reaction occurs in the body. Many researchers think that this type of oxidizing over a lifetime produces the aging of our tissues.

Fortunately, your body produces several enzymes that protect your tissues against damage from oxygen and other radicals. In addition to these enzymes, your body uses vitamin C, beta-carotene, vitamin E, and vitamin A to intercept (quench) oxygen radicals and convert them into harmless substances. Several longitudinal studies, particularly ones done in Finland and in Basel, Switzerland, provide evidence that people who have a high intake of vitamin C and beta-carotene and who maintain appreciable blood levels of these nutrients through their lives have significantly lower risk of cancer than other people.

Protective Ingredient No. 1: Vitamin C

Vitamin C is present in many complex carbohydrate foods, such as citrus fruits, tomatoes, strawberries, potatoes, broccoli, Brussels sprouts, green peppers, spinach, turnips, cantaloupes, and kiwis.

Vitamin C helps prevent environmentally induced cancer in various ways. For example, it quenches free radicals and converts them into harmless substances that are easily eliminated. It also decreases the chance that various free radicals will bind to the genetic material of your cells; in that way it protects your genes from undergoing cancerous changes. Vitamin C also helps prevent cancer by blocking the formation of nitrosamines in your stomach, intestines, bladder, and other tissues. Nitrosamines are carcinogenic. They result mainly from eating cold cuts and bacon, which contain nitrite salts and nitrate salts. There is now also nitrate in the soils and drinking water as a result of the wide use of nitrate fertilizers. Obviously, you cannot stop eating foods grown from the soil or drinking water, but you can increase your consumption of foods containing vitamin C, thus reducing the likelihood that your body will manufacture these dangerous, cancer-causing chemicals.

Also, your liver relies heavily on vitamin C to help detoxify environmental toxins, drugs, and alcohol, all of which can damage your genes.

Vitamin C boosts your body's overall immune system by increasing the ability of your white blood cells to attack and destroy invading viruses and microorganisms. Research has taught us that cancer prevention and a healthy immune system go hand in hand.

Protective Ingredient No. 2: Vitamin E
Vitamin E is another anti-cancer protective nutrient that quenches free radicals in your body. It is found in wheat germ, which is an excellent complex carbohydrate food.

Protective Ingredient No. 3: Beta-Carotene
The orange/yellow pigment that produces the characteristic coloring of carrots, squash, apricots, peaches, nectarines, cantaloupes, and sweet potatoes is the anti-cancer protective nutrient known as beta-carotene. Beta-carotene is also found in green leafy vegetables and broccoli. Like vitamin C, beta-carotene is a very powerful quencher of free radicals, especially on the surface of such organs as the lungs and stomach and along the bodily passages. This action reduces the risk of lung cancer and stomach cancer. It also provides some protection against ovarian, breast, uterine, cervical, prostate, oral cavity, bladder, and throat cancer. Numerous research papers now substantiate the claim that people who regularly eat food high in beta-carotene and vitamin C tend to have the lowest overall cancer risk in most populations.

Protective Ingredient No. 4: Indole Rings
Cruciferous vegetables, including Brussels sprouts, cabbage, cauliflower, broccoli, and turnips, contain an anti-cancer ingredient known as *indole rings.* Indole rings stimulate detoxification centers within your body cells. These detoxification centers deactivate

and neutralize many environmental toxins before they can be converted into volatile free radicals. Research studies have shown that people who eat cruciferous vegetables have a lower risk of developing many types of cancer.

Protective Ingredient No. 5: Fiber

There is another way that complex carbohydrates protect you against cancer, particularly colon cancer. As you may already know, the occurrence rate of colon cancer makes it the second major type of cancer in our society.

The fiber found in complex carbohydrate foods has been found to be so important to general health that we have given fiber its own section. Here we will just mention that the fiber found in wheat bran, corn bran, and rice bran will help reduce your risk of colon cancer. These brans are available in a variety of foods, such as high-fiber breakfast cereal, whole wheat bread, whole wheat biscuits, corn on the cob, popcorn, puffed corn cereals, brown rice, and rice crackers.

Exhibit 2-2
Sources of Anti-Cancer Protective Nutrients

Vitamin C:	citrus fruit, tomatoes, potatoes, broccoli, Brussels sprouts, green peppers, spinach, turnips, cantaloupes, kiwis
Vitamin E:	wheat germ
Beta-carotene:	carrots, apricots, sweet potatoes, broccoli, squash, peaches, green leafy vegetables
Cruciferous vegetables:	cabbage, cauliflower, Brussels sprouts, broccoli, turnips
Fiber:	wheat bran, corn bran, rice bran

There is no question that your body is designed to use complex carbohydrates as its main source of nutrition. Fruits, vegetables, rice, pasta, bread, low-fat biscuits, high-fiber breakfast cereals, peas, beans, jams, and broth soups with noodles, rice, or vegetables should make up 55 to 65 percent of your daily calories if you want to control your weight, extend your life, increase your energy and overall fitness, and protect yourself against cancer and heart disease. The next step in the Winning Weigh will show you how to reach that goal, but start right now to use what you have learned to improve your eating habits.

Starting Right Now . . .

1. Begin replacing high-fat foods with the life-enhancing complex carbohydrate foods we have listed in this chapter.
    a. Instead of putting butter or margarine on toast or a bagel, use jam. Although jams contain some white sugar, most jams are made from whole fruits and contain added fiber (pectin and gum fiber).
    b. Instead of high-fat potato chips and dip, nacho chips, or any fried treat of this kind, try these complex carbohydrate alternatives:
        (i) low-fat biscuits, such as melba toast, dipped in salsa sauce
        (ii) baked pretzels dipped into salsa sauce or mustard
        (iii) popcorn with no added butter or high-fat toppings (an air popper is best)
    c. As a snack between meals, choose
        (i) fruit
        (ii) raisins or any other dried fruits
        (iii) low-fat bran muffin
        (iv) plain bagel or bagel with jam
        (v) carrot sticks

2. Don't be afraid to eat more starchy carbohydrates, such as bread, pasta, rice, and potatoes. However, do not smother them in fats. Instead, use whole fruit jam on bread, tomato sauce on pasta, and low-fat yogurt on potatoes or, better still, have the baked potato naked or with just pepper.
3. When you drink fruit juice, add three parts water to one part juice. Fruit juices are too concentrated with simple sugars to be taken straight up.
4. Whenever possible, eat complex carbohydrate foods high in anti-cancer nutrients. Try to have at least one complex carbohydrate that contains anti-cancer nutrients at every meal.
5. When you eat complex carbohydrate foods, envision the five ways they can help you lose weight if this has been a problem for you:
   a. They have half as many calories as the same amount of fat.
   b. You don't absorb 10 to 20 percent of their calories.
   c. You burn more calories to digest them (thermogenesis).
   d. They make you feel full sooner.
   e. They prime your body for burning fat.
6. Fill out the Wellness Planner on complex carbohydrates, page 306.

Fiber

In the previous section, we said that complex carbohydrates are the only sources of dietary fiber. Dietary fiber is emerging as a vital nutritional ingredient in wellness. It can help prevent many cancers, cardiovascular diseases, and excess weight gain. Unfortunately, most people in North America are eating only a third of the amount of fiber they need.

In response to a growing public awareness of the importance of fiber, the food industry has introduced an increasing number of high-fiber breakfast cereals, crackers, and other products. This awareness can be directly attributed to the research pioneered by Doctors Burkitt and Trowell, who suggested that the Africans' high-fiber diet was directly linked to their strong resistance to cancer, diabetes, heart disease, strokes, hemorrhoids, and varicose veins. This research sparked the interest of other scientists, who investigated the specific health benefits of dietary fiber. In the past 15 years, a wealth of knowledge has grown out of their efforts.

The Nature of Fiber

Where exactly do we find fiber in our daily diet? Almost all unprocessed foods derived from plants contain fiber. In contrast, no food of animal origin contains fiber. There is no fiber in red meat, poultry, fish, dairy products, or eggs.

Ironically, the importance of fiber is that we cannot digest it. Fiber is really nothing more than long, branching chains of complex carbohydrates. These carbohydrates are strung together in such a peculiar arrangement that our digestive systems are unable to break them apart. Although some fiber is metabolized by bacteria in the large intestine, much of it passes through the entire length of our intestines almost unaltered. It makes up the bulk of our fecal matter and plays an essential role in maintaining the health of the intestinal tract.

Unfortunately, in the last century we have learned to prefer our food, particularly our grains, heavily refined. As a result, many of us suffer the consequences of fiber deficiency, setting ourselves up for heart disease, excess weight gain, and colon and rectal problems. Over the last 100 years, for example, our increasingly high-fat, low-fiber diet has made colon-rectal cancer the leading cancer killer when the statistics for men and women are combined.

The Winning Weigh nutritional program puts a heavy emphasis on fiber, but we won't ask you to eat sawdust shavings at every meal. You may equate fiber with dry, tasteless bran cereals instead of with something positive and flavorful. It's time for you to change that attitude. Bran fiber is beneficial to your health, but so is the fiber found in fruits, vegetables, legumes, and oats. In fact, these different types of fiber contribute to your health in different ways.

Scientists have discovered many different types of fiber and have given them highly technical names like pectin, guar gum, lignin, cellulose, and hemi-cellulose. We have simplified these fibers into two groups according to their effects in your body: cholesterol crunchers and colon cleaners. Some foods contain a lot of cholesterol cruncher fiber, which helps to lower high blood cholesterol and to regulate blood sugar levels. Other foods contain more colon cleaner fiber, which helps protect against cancer of the colon and rectum, irritable bowel syndrome, and many related conditions.

Cholesterol Crunchers

Some complex carbohydrates contain fiber that can lower elevated blood cholesterol levels. As everyone knows by now, elevated cholesterol can reduce the diameter of your arteries over time. Constricted arteries can lead to heart attacks, strokes, and kidney failure. Cardiovascular diseases such as these account for approximately 50 percent of all the deaths in our society. Keeping your cholesterol down now can prevent you from adding to this statistic later.

Some complex carbohydrates contain a type of fiber that clings to cholesterol in the intestinal tract like a magnet and stops it from being absorbed into the bloodstream where it can do damage. Instead, these cholesterol crunchers drag cholesterol through the large bowel and eliminate it in the feces. They eliminate bile acids in the same way.

After a meal, bile acids are secreted by the gallbladder to aid in fat digestion. These bile acids tend to be reabsorbed into the body and converted into cholesterol by the liver. The presence of cholesterol crunchers in the intestine stops the absorption of bile acids into the body and promotes their elimination in the feces as well.

An average fasting blood cholesterol level for North Americans is approximately 225 mg percent. In a society where 50 percent of people die from cardiovascular disease, the average cholesterol level is obviously not a good level to maintain. To be safe, you should work to get your blood cholesterol level below 200 mg percent. The safest range seems to be between 150 and 160 mg percent.

If your fasting blood cholesterol level is 260 mg percent, you are only 9 percent above the average, but that 9 percent increase will double your risk of heart attack. By simply eating 15 grams (one tablespoon) of oat bran every day, you can reduce the 260 mg percent to 225, cutting your risk in half again. Studies have proven that adding cholesterol crunchers to your daily diet can lower blood cholesterol levels by 10 to 15 percent. For some people, lowering the level by this much can mean the difference between life and death. Given the fact that heart attacks and other cardiovascular diseases are responsible for approximately 50 percent of deaths each year in North America, getting enough cholesterol crunchers in your diet is vital.

Cholesterol crunchers also help prevent your body from manufacturing more cholesterol. Eating foods high in fat triggers the production of bile acids. These bile acids can be reabsorbed into the body and converted into cholesterol. Cholesterol crunchers cling to the bile acids in the intestinal tract and drag them out of the body as part of the feces **before** they can be converted into cholesterol.

Cholesterol crunchers also slow down the rate at which carbohydrates in the intestinal tract are absorbed into the bloodstream. Less complex carbohydrates, such as sugar and honey, are absorbed into your bloodstream very quickly, which puts undue stress on your liver and pancreas. Cholesterol crunchers help to regulate blood sugar levels.

Finally, cholesterol crunchers make you feel full, so they discourage you from overeating. Most of us tend to eat until we feel a sense of satisfaction (satiety). Cholesterol crunchers will produce a feeling of satiety faster than any other food except fat (which is not good for you). To prove this to yourself, eat two apples, a banana, or a grapefruit (about 120 calories) the next time you feel hungry between meals. By eating these satiety-producing fruits, you will almost immediately overcome the powerful temptation to eat sweet or rich foods. If you eat less, you lower your intake of calories.

Feeling hungry and deprived is not the way to achieve long-term wellness. High-fiber foods are high-satisfaction foods. Fresh fruit, pumpernickel and rye bread, popcorn, pita bread, and baked bagels are good alternatives to high-fat, high-calorie junk foods. These high-fiber foods will satisfy your psychological investment in eating.

Exhibit 2–3
Foods High in Cholesterol Crunchers

The complex carbohydrates that contain the richest supply of cholesterol cruncher fiber are

1. oat bran, oatmeal, and oats
2. psyllium husk fiber (Metamucil®)
3. apples, peaches, pears, and plums
4. berries (strawberries, raspberries, blackberries, boysenberries, etc.), but not cherries
5. white rind of citrus fruits (the white stuff under the skin of oranges, grapefruits, tangerines, etc.)
6. carrots and potatoes
7. peas and beans, especially chick-peas and kidney beans
8. pumpernickel bread

"Apples, peaches, pears, and plums / Tell me when your birthday comes." Say this childhood rhyme three times, and you'll never forget which fruits are high in cholesterol crunchers.

Colon Cleaners

Colon cleaners form the second family of fibers in the Winning Weigh nutritional program. Like cholesterol crunchers, colon cleaners are not digested or absorbed in the intestinal tract. However, they play a different role than cholesterol crunchers in the large intestines.

It has been known for some time that protein foods containing nitrates and nitrites, such as bacon, pepperoni, salami, hot dogs, most packaged meats, and most cold cuts, encourage the development of cancer in the colon and rectum. When the protein in these processed meats reacts with the nitrate and nitrite preservatives during digestion, carcinogenic nitrosamines are formed. These nitrosamine chemicals are only one type of cancer-causing agent against which the body must defend itself daily.

When you eat fats, your liver and gallbladder secrete bile acids into the intestine. Bile acids that are not absorbed back into the body as cholesterol remain in the intestinal tract. These can be converted into cancer-causing agents by the bacteria that line the large intestine. In this way, a diet that is high in fats contributes to the development of colon cancer.

As you may already know, the occurrence rate of colon cancer makes it the second major type of cancer in our society. Once you pass the age of 40, your risk of incurring colon cancer increases 40-fold over the next 40 years. This rapid increase in the incidence of colon cancer with age doesn't occur in parts of the world where less fats and more complex carbohydrates, especially whole grains and beans, are eaten.

Colon cleaners help protect you from these and other carcinogens in two ways.

1. **Colon cleaners dilute the levels of cancer-causing agents in your intestinal tract.**

Acting like a sponge, colon cleaners soak up water in the intestinal tract. As a result, the fecal matter being formed in the intestinal tract has a high water content, which dilutes the concentration of cancer-causing agents. Generally, the higher the concentration of cancer-causing agents, the greater the likelihood that they will cause genetic damage to the cells that line your colon and rectum.

2. **Colon cleaners move fecal matter quickly through your intestinal tract.**

The sponge-like colon cleaners absorb water, expanding the bulk of fecal matter. This expansion exerts physical pressure against the inside walls of the intestinal tract, which in turn stimulates synchronized contractions of the muscular layers of the intestinal walls. These muscular contractions propel the fecal matter through the intestinal tract and out of the body. This decreases the time during which your intestines, colon, and rectum are exposed to cancer-causing agents. By absorbing water, colon cleaner fiber also dilutes toxic wastes and cancer radicals and enables the body to more quickly eliminate them.

To improve the function of colon cleaners, you must drink enough water to take advantage of their sponge-like behavior. Six to eight (8 oz) glasses of water every day is enough. You should also be sure to have frequent bowel movements. One per day is excellent; five per week is acceptable; three or less is dangerous. An additional benefit is that the high water content of stools formed by colon cleaners makes them soft and easy to eliminate from the body. They require minimal straining and are therefore less likely to cause hemorrhoids and varicose veins. (You will know your stools are sufficiently high in water content if they float.) Rock-hard, pellet-like stools are solid evidence that you lack sufficient colon cleaner fiber to protect you from one of the most common life-threatening cancers of our day – one that is clearly related to diet.

Foods High in Colon Cleaners

Complex carbohydrate foods that are loaded with colon cleaner fiber include wheat bran, corn bran, and rice bran. These brans are available in a variety of foods, such as high-fiber breakfast cereal, whole wheat bread, whole wheat biscuits, corn on the cob, popcorn, puffed corn cereals, brown rice, and rice crackers. Some additional sources of colon cleaner fiber include red kidney beans, chick-peas, and psyllium husk fiber (the main ingredient in Metamucil®). The main sources of colon cleaners are listed in Exhibit 2-4.

Exhibit 2-4
Sources of Colon Cleaners

Whole grain products
Wheat bran, including whole wheat products and bran cereals
Rice bran, including brown rice, puffed rice, and whole rice crackers
Corn bran, including corn, popcorn, cornmeal, and corn flakes
Peas and beans (especially chick-peas and kidney beans)
High-fiber breakfast cereals (except oatmeal)
Psyllium husk fiber (Metamucil®)

Fiber in Your Diet

Keeping track of the amount of fiber you eat is easy on the Winning Weigh. We have provided a fiber scoreboard on page 293 that assigns points according to the fiber content of common foods. A medium apple, for example, has one point. In order to take full advantage of colon cleaners and cholesterol crunchers, you should eat 8 to 15 fiber points from a variety of foods every day. On page 94, we also give you the recipe for the Winning Weigh Fiber Mixture, made of oat bran, wheat bran, and wheat germ. This mixture will meet your daily needs for both colon cleaners and cholesterol crunchers.

We will discuss the practicalities of using the Fiber Scoreboard and Fiber Mixture in Step 3. In the meantime, drink plenty of water to optimize the benefits of fiber and choose foods that are high in fiber.

Exhibit 2–5
Good Sources of Fiber

High in Fiber	Low in Fiber
Whole wheat flour, rye, pumpernickel, or other dark breads	White bread, white flour products
Whole wheat or spinach noodles	White flour noodles
Brown rice	White rice
Apples, peaches, pears, plums citrus fruits, berries, raisins, whole-fruit jams	Grapes, cherries, bananas, melons
Beans and peas	
Carrots, potatoes, cauliflower, Brussels sprouts, cabbage, yams, beets	Cucumbers, lettuce
Fig Newtons, popcorn, baked pita, chips, fruit salad	Sherbet, angel food cake, chef's salad

Starting Right Now . . .

1. As you eat foods high in cholesterol crunchers, imagine that they are magnets, dragging the cholesterol and saturated fats through your intestinal tract and out of your body.

2. As you eat foods high in colon cleaners, envision the food as a vacuum cleaner, sucking the carcinogens and other toxins from the walls of your bowels.

3. Choose foods that are high in fiber, both colon cleaners and cholesterol crunchers.

4. If you are indulging in a high-cholesterol food, be sure to eat a food high in cholesterol crunchers at the same time. This combination reduces the amount of cholesterol that gets absorbed into your bloodstream.

5. Drink six to eight glasses of water every day. Plenty of water is necessary for colon cleaners to work at their optimal potential.

6. Make sure you are having a bowel movement at least five times a week. Also make sure your stools float. If they do not, drink more water. Pay attention to how your bowel movements are affected by your diet. Get to know your own body rhythms.

7. Eat wheat germ often. It is high in vitamin E and fiber. Sprinkle it on cereal, mix it into yogurt, or add it to foods such as muffins. You can also get it in the Winning Weigh Fiber Mixture (see p. 94)

8. Try to eat naturally occurring complex carbohydrate foods instead of modified ones. For example, eat brown rice instead of white rice and whole wheat bread instead of white bread.

9. Become aware of your body's sense of fullness and satisfaction after a high-fiber breakfast or snack. Compare how you feel after a breakfast of oatmeal or bran cereal to how you feel after a low-fiber breakfast of bacon and eggs. You are much less likely to crave a mid-morning snack.

10. Do not eat processed meats, including hot dogs, bacon, pepperoni, salami, most packaged meats, and most cold cuts. Not only are they full of saturated fats, but they are full of cancer-causing preservatives.

11. In the Wellness Planner (p. 307), write a list of the high-fiber foods that you are going to start eating more often. Be sure to include both cholesterol crunchers and colon cleaners.

Fats

The verdict on dietary fat is in: our eating habits are killing us. The diet of the average North American consists of up to 43 percent fat. This astronomical level is the **number one nutritional cause of heart attack, stroke, certain types of cancer, and obesity.** And that's no exaggeration! It's no wonder that everywhere you turn health authorities are telling you to cut back on the amount of fat you eat. For example, the American Heart Association, the American Cancer Association, the Diabetic Association, and the National Institute of Health (NIH) have, for a long time, strongly recommended reducing your fat intake.

On the other hand, you don't have to be paranoid about fat. It's essential to eat some fat every day to stay healthy. Some types of fat, such as the Omega 3 fats found in fish, help protect you from heart disease, stroke, and various cancers. The predominant fat found in olive oil and peanut oil provides similar benefits.

How Much Fat Is Enough?

The question is, how much fat is enough? Some nutrition fanatics insist that you should eat nothing but grains, vegetables, tofu, and brewers' yeast, thus limiting your total fat intake to only 10 to 15 percent of your total daily calories. However, this type of program is very difficult to follow and is unnecessarily restrictive for 90 to 95 percent of the population. A growing body of evidence indicates that you can get as much as 20 to 25 percent of your total calories from fat without promoting cardiovascular disease, cancer, or obesity. However, if you have a high risk of cardiovascular disease, you would be wise to restrict your fat intake to 20 percent of your calories or less.

Some health authorities, such as the Heart Association, allow 30 percent of your total calories to come from fat. Although this percentage is not ideal, they think that most people would be unwilling to change their eating habits more than that. They figure that 30 percent fat is better than the 43 percent that most North Americans now ingest.

The level of cholesterol in your blood will probably decrease if you reduce your fat intake to 30 percent. However, many people will not see dramatic results until they cut back to 20 to 25 percent. That extra 5 to 10 percent can make a big difference. We have many patients who were once overweight with high blood pressure, but who are now slim, fit, and healthy. They have proven that getting no more that 25 percent of their total calories from fat is practical and painless.

However, the question of how much fat is enough is more complicated than determining the ideal total intake. The fat in your diet is made up of four different types, or families: saturated fats, polyunsaturated fats, monounsaturated fats, and Omega 3 fats (a special type of polyunsaturated fat). You need the proper amount of each family of fat because each affects your health and risk of disease in different ways. ***You will reach the most healthy balance if you get approximately one-third of your fat calories from saturated fats, one-third from monounsaturated fats, and one-third from polyunsaturated and Omega 3 fats.***

You will not need to become a food faddist or a nutritional evangelist. You can enjoy a wide variety of foods without counting a single calorie or performing a single calculation. Using the Winning Weigh nutritional system, ***sticking to a diet of 20 to 25 percent total fat intake, properly balanced between the different types of fat, is very practical and easy to do on a long-term basis.***

The Dangers of Too Much Fat

Many health-conscious people are very concerned about white sugar in their diets. They fail to recognize that ***excess fat consumption*** is the most serious nutritional health problem in North America today, much more serious than sugar. Pastries for dessert, large slabs of butter melting over a baked potato, bacon and eggs for breakfast, cheddar cheese smothering a plate of nachos, processed meats from the local deli: these high-fat foods are the primary dietary killers in our society today. They clog up your arteries, increasing your chances of heart attacks, angina, and strokes. They can also overstimulate your hormonal system, increasing your risk of cancers of the reproductive organs (breasts, ovaries, cervix, and prostate). Cancer researchers have known for a long time now that excess dietary fat is a powerful promoter of many forms of cancer, including colon and rectal cancer.

Fifty percent of people in North America die of heart disease and related cardiovascular problems. Approximately another 20 percent die of cancer. And the cancers that kill the most people – lung, breast, colon/rectal, and reproductive organ cancers – are primarily related to lifestyle. That means you can decrease your chances of getting these diseases by changing the moment-by-moment decisions you make.

We are not overstating these dangers. People now know that smoking can lead to lung cancer. Fewer people seem to realize that the research linking a high-fat diet (particularly a diet high in saturated fat) with cancer is also too convincing to be ignored. The consensus in the medical field is that eating too much fat is the ***major risk factor*** for most diet-related disease. The scientific evidence is so convincing that the Surgeon General of the United States, always extremely conservative, released a Report on Nutrition and Health in July 1988 presenting its first comprehensive review of the scientific evidence that links diet to chronic disease. This report recognizes that the most common nutrition-related problems and conditions among people in the United States are due to obesity and unbalanced diets. It identifies reducing the consumption of fat, especially of saturated fat, as the ***primary dietary priority*** for improving overall health:

> Dietary fat is the single most important dietary factor that is linked to degenerative diseases, especially saturated fat.

Eating Fat Makes You Fat

Not only is eating a lot of fat related directly to heart disease and some cancers, but it is the major reason for becoming overweight. Your body stores fat very efficiently. Digesting, absorbing, transporting, and storing the fat you eat uses up only 7 percent of its initial calories. In other words, your body delivers the fat from your diet and stores it in your fat cells with an efficiency rate of **93 percent.** So, simply stated, when you eat fat, you get fat, especially if you have a slow metabolism.

As a general rule, you can change the number of fat cells in your body only until you are about 19 years old. After that, you will have the same number of fat cells for the rest of your life, unless you gain a tremendous amount of weight. Consequently, most adults *could* remain at the same weight as they were at 19 years of age. In fact, this is the weight that bodies are programmed to be.

Adults in North America gain an average of one to two pounds every year after the age of 25. So by the age of 50, they are 25 to 50 pounds overweight. Their fat cells, rather than increasing in number, become larger. In fact, fat cells can expand in size almost indefinitely. However, a positive wellness program such as the Winning Weigh can help you maintain the weight you were when you were 19 years old.

What if you were overweight at 19? Because of your higher number of fat cells, you will always have a more difficult time looking lean. However, if you were overweight at 19, following a wellness program will still make you look and feel better. Just try not to feel obsessed with your weight. Begin eating more complex carbohydrates, eat less fat, and just watch what happens. You'll love the improvement.

Saturated Fat

Each of the four families of fat plays its own role in determining your state of health and risk of disease. Their powerful influences on your body's metabolism can either promote or discourage inflammatory conditions, heart attacks, high blood pressure, and cancer. The proper balance of these four families of fat in your diet is an essential component of any wellness program.

Let's look first at the most dangerous family of dietary fat–saturated fats. On the Winning Weigh diet system, roughly one-third of your total fat intake is in saturated fats. Sticking to this guideline is probably the most important step you can take in preventing cardiovascular diseases. Furthermore, most obesity is the result of eating foods containing calorie-rich saturated fats.

Exhibit 2–6
Foods High in Saturated Fat

Sour cream, butter, whole milk, cream, ice cream

Cheese that is more than 18% milk fat (e.g., cheddar cheese, blue, brick, colby, cream, muenster, port du salut)

Egg yolks

Marbled red meats (steak), processed luncheon meats (hot dogs, salami, bologna, prosciutto, corned beef, pastrami, spare ribs, bacon), organ meats (liver, kidney)

Chocolate (cocoa butter), coconut oil

Baked goods and candy made from palm oil or palm kernel oil

Saturated Fat and Cholesterol

Saturated fats interact with cholesterol to give you double trouble. Surprisingly, it's not necessarily the cholesterol in food that elevates your blood cholesterol levels. In fact, up to two-thirds of the cholesterol in your body is produced by your liver. Only one-third comes from the cholesterol you eat.

Usually, **elevated blood cholesterol is a result of eating too much saturated fat.** When you eat saturated fat, it is absorbed from your intestines. Then, most of it is carried to your liver, which it stimulates to produce cholesterol. So if you eat a food that is high in saturated fat, your body responds by turning on the cholesterol-manufacturing plant in your liver. And the more saturated fat you eat, the more cholesterol your liver produces.

Coconut oil and palm oil, used in commercially-made baked goods, don't contain any cholesterol at all, but they are heavily loaded with saturated fat. In fact, it's their saturated fat content that makes them ideal for baking: they are very stable when heated to high temperatures. When these saturated fats enter your body as part of cookies, pie crust, and other pastries, they are transported to your liver where they stimulate cholesterol production.

Chocolate can have the same effect. It contains no cholesterol but, because of its high saturated fat content, it may increase the level of cholesterol in your blood. Cholesterol builds up in your body even though you haven't eaten any. So beware of foods advertised as being cholesterol-free – this doesn't mean they won't increase the level of cholesterol in your blood.

The situation is worse if you eat foods that contain high levels of saturated fat *and* cholesterol. These foods really clog your arteries in a hurry. Saturated fat and cholesterol are only found together in foods of animal origin. The trick to avoiding this double whammy is to eat low-fat, low-cholesterol dairy products, which still provide you with calcium, vitamin D, and protein. And you should eat

Exhibit 2–7
A Double Whammy:
Foods High in Saturated Fat and Cholesterol

Whole milk products (chocolate milk, whole milk yogurt, heavy cream)
High-fat cheeses, ice cream, butter
Mayonnaise, eggs yolks (not egg whites)
Organ meats (liver, brains, sweetbreads, kidney, and heart), red meats (beef, pork, untrimmed lamb and veal), sausage, bacon, cold cuts

chicken, turkey, Cornish hen, lean veal, and fish instead of high-fat meat products. These provide additional vitamin B_{12} and iron.

How Your Body Handles Cholesterol

So how does cholesterol contribute to the threat of heart disease, strokes, and certain types of cancer? The answer is really quite remarkable. One of your liver's primary objectives is to transport the saturated fat you have eaten to other tissues of the body. This task is not an easy one because fats can't dissolve in your bloodstream. (You know the saying, "Oil and water don't mix.") The liver must therefore repackage the fat with other more dissolvable substances before it can travel through your bloodstream: it builds, in effect, a miniature "shuttle bus." The outer frame of the shuttle bus is made up of protein and the inside is filled with saturated fat and cholesterol.

Once the bus is full, it is sealed and shipped out of the liver to enter the bloodstream. The outer protein shell of the bus allows part of the fat and cholesterol to dissolve and float freely. As the shuttle bus passes by muscles, it opens its doors and allows some fat to be taken up. As a rule, when your muscles are not working vigorously, they prefer to burn fat, thus preserving their stores of carbohydrates for use as high-octane fuel during strenuous exercise. (Your heart muscle in particular likes to burn fat for energy.) The shuttle bus eventually transports any additional saturated fat throughout your bloodstream to be stored in your fat cells. This is how your fat cells become enlarged and you begin to look fat.

But what about the cholesterol in the shuttle bus? It is also delivered to your body cells. In the adrenal glands, cholesterol is used to make hormones such as cortisone. In the ovaries, it is used to make estrogen and progesterone. In the male testes, it is the building block of the male hormone testosterone. Cholesterol is also used to build bile acids, vitamin D, and part of the fatty, waxy membrane around the outside of every body cell.

Exhibit 2-8
Saturated Fat and Cholesterol in Your Body

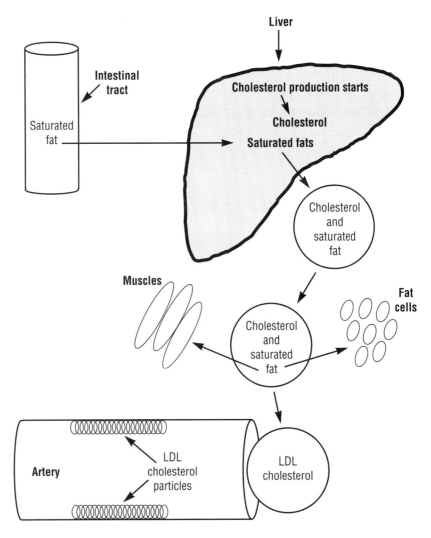

When you eat saturated fat, your liver starts producing cholesterol. Cholesterol and saturated fat travel through the bloodstream together. Much of the saturated fat is picked up by fat cells and muscles, where it is stored as fat or burned for energy. The remaining particles left behind in the bloodstream become the LDL cholesterol particles. These tend to narrow arteries by clinging to the artery wall.

So far so good – your body needs a certain amount of cholesterol to remain healthy. However, when you consume a diet high in saturated fat and/or cholesterol, the shuttle buses transport more cholesterol than your body cells require for their normal functions. In this situation, the shuttle bus doors can open and allow excess cholesterol to exit into the bloodstream, where it becomes stuck to the inside linings of the blood vessel walls. This process causes the blood vessels to narrow, eventually restricting the circulation of blood.

This narrowing process, known as **atherosclerosis** (hardening of the arteries), is the major contributing cause of heart disease, stroke, and related cardiovascular diseases. Less blood and oxygen can circulate to the heart muscle, resulting in an angina episode or a heart attack. In the brain, these narrowed vessels become rigid, losing their elasticity. Then they are more easily ruptured, resulting in a stroke.

The Big Plaque Attack

The cholesterol that gets laid down in your arteries from the cholesterol shuttle bus forms the main component of arterial plaque. As the arterial plaque thickens over your lifetime, your heart arteries (coronary arteries) and other arteries become narrower. Once an artery is almost completely obstructed by arterial plaque, you become a prime candidate for a heart attack, stroke, or even kidney failure. Unfortunately, arterial narrowing due to arterial plaque is completely invisible and painless until the final stages. That is why death by heart attack or stroke can happen suddenly, with no warning signs.

It is, of course, human nature not to pay attention to things that we can't see or feel. The Dental Association has a relatively easy job convincing us to floss and brush our teeth to prevent the build-up of dental plaque. We can feel plaque on our teeth. But what about plaque in our arteries? We can't see or feel that.

Yet no one has ***ever*** died because of dental plaque on their teeth. Arterial plaque, on the other hand, is life-threatening. Fifty percent of North Americans die of cardiovascular diseases, most of them as a result of obstructed and rigid arteries. Just because you can't see it or feel it doesn't mean you should ignore it. If you are lucky, you will get advance warning of the build-up of arterial plaque – the squeezing chest and arm pain of angina. Unfortunately, for 25 percent of the people with advanced blood-vessel narrowing, sudden death by heart attack is their first and last symptom of heart disease.

To make matters worse, some evidence suggests that excess cholesterol delivered to your fat tissues, adrenal glands, ovaries, and testes may overstimulate the production of certain hormones and produce abnormally formed hormones. Imbalances in these reproductive hormones have been associated with the increased risk of breast cancer, prostate cancer, and other cancers of the reproductive organs.

In a nutshell, eating foods high in saturated fat forces the liver to manufacture large quantities of cholesterol. Any excess cholesterol travelling through the bloodstream sticks to the inside walls of your arteries. Cumulative lifetime narrowing of the arteries is one of the main reasons why you can feel fine one minute and die of a heart attack the next. It's the old story of the straw that broke the camel's back: every mouthful of saturated fat that you eat adds another layer of arterial plaque. One day the artery may be completely obstructed. How long do you plan to wait before you appreciate the full impact that high-fat foods have on your life expectancy?

The Good Guys and the Bad Guys

Now the story gets more complicated – not all cholesterol contributes to the hardening of your arteries. Up to this point, we have been discussing only the LDL cholesterol shuttle bus. The liver also makes an **HDL** cholesterol shuttle bus, which it also releases to the bloodstream. This HDL cholesterol shuttle bus actually **vacuums** up deposits of LDL cholesterol from your artery walls and carries it back to your liver. There it can be used for other purposes, such as producing bile acids. (Of course, if you are still eating foods high in saturated fats and cholesterol, your liver will have too much cholesterol already and will just send it back out to your arteries again.)

Studies have shown that people with high levels of HDL cholesterol (the good guys) and low levels of LDL cholesterol (the bad guys) are much less likely to develop heart attacks or advanced stages of atherosclerosis. Some recent studies have even confirmed that raising your levels of HDL cholesterol can actually reverse the hardening of your arteries that has already occurred.

Certainly, the ratio of your LDL to HDL cholesterol levels can tell your doctor a lot about your present chances of developing cardiovascular disease. So next time you are getting some blood work done, ask to see where you stand. But even if your LDL to HDL ratio is low, remember that it is easier to cut back on saturated fat and cholesterol now than to wait until the damage is already done.

Play It Smart, Play It Safe

The only real way to play it safe when it comes to eating saturated fat and LDL cholesterol is to keep your consumption within the boundaries set by our Winning Weigh nutritional system. Along with the Winning Weigh exercise programs, this will help keep your saturated fat and LDL cholesterol levels down, while you try to increase your level of HDL cholesterol through aerobic exercise, eating more fish, and using olive oil instead of other types of fat.

You won't have to sit up at night calculating your saturated fat and cholesterol intake. We have formulated the program to allow you to enjoy meat, fish, fowl, and dairy products without paying the price of obesity, heart disease, stroke, or lifestyle-related cancer. The Winning Weigh program will help to prevent excess LDL cholesterol from building up in your system while you enjoy a variety of animal-based protein foods. It is this type of flexibility that makes the Winning Weigh practical, easy to implement, and agreeable.

Exhibit 2–9
Sources of Saturated Fat
in the Winning Weigh Nutritional Program

- Chicken, turkey, and Cornish hens
- Lean veal or beef occasionally
- Cheese that is under 10% milk fat (M.F.)
- Skim milk
- Other low-fat dairy products

Polyunsaturated Fats

Polyunsaturated fats are an essential ingredient for good health. Early studies showed that corn oil, a substance high in polyunsaturated fats, could lower blood cholesterol levels. However, we realize today that polyunsaturated oils may actually present more danger to your health than benefit. First of all, they contain many unstable double bonds that allow them to be easily converted into free radicals. Animal studies have shown that a diet rich in polyunsaturated fats increases the incidence of spontaneous tumor development quite markedly.

A second problem develops from the tendency of polyunsaturated fats to become the building block of a chemical called ***thromboxane***. Thromboxane encourages your blood platelets to stick together more readily than they normally do, resulting in clogged arteries and inflammation in the artery walls. In addition, thromboxane encourages arteries to go into spasm, resulting in further narrowing.

If you want to keep your blood vessels open and minimize your risk of heart disease or stroke, you need to try to keep the amount of thromboxane you produce from polyunsaturated fats low. Avoid corn oil, sunflower seed oil, safflower oil, and soybean oil, and the products made from them. Instead, choose oils that are high in monounsaturated fats – olive oil, peanut oil, and canola oil.

Exhibit 2-10
Avoid Foods High in Polyunsaturated Fat

Most vegetable oils (including corn oil, sunflower seed oil, soybean oil, and safflower oil)

Partially hydrogenated foods, such as margarine, shortening, and processed peanut butter

An Extra Danger: Partially Hydrogenated Foods

Partially hydrogenated foods, such as margarine, vegetable shortening, and processed peanut butter, can be especially dangerous. These foods are made from polyunsaturated fats that have been made more saturated. Although this process makes them solid and therefore easier to spread, your body has difficulty using partially hydrogenated polyunsaturated fats; it does not know what they are.

Recent studies have demonstrated that hydrogenated fats raise cholesterol levels, as if you were eating saturated fats. These fats also encourage the formation of thromboxane and other potentially harmful substances. All in all, they are best avoided.

Monounsaturated Fats

We have discussed the first two families of fats: saturated fats, found primarily in dairy and meat products, and polyunsaturated fats, found in most vegetable oils. The third family is composed of monounsaturated fats, found mainly in olive oil, peanut oil, and canola oil. These fats help lower cholesterol but are much more stable than polyunsaturated fats when exposed to heat, air, and light. They are not easily converted into free radicals.

Mediterranean and Oriental civilizations have relied on olive oil and peanut oil as their main sources of dietary fat for thousands of years. People from these cultures have less risk of heart disease and certain forms of cancer than North Americans in general. Knowledge about the benefits of these oils has been passed down through the generations in Mediterranean and Oriental civilizations. Because olive oil and peanut oil have been used in the human diet for centuries without ill effects, we know they are safe.

We know less about rapeseed oil, commonly known as canola oil, because people have just begun to use it recently. However, recent research suggests that it provides the same benefits as olive oil and peanut oil do.

Some new evidence suggests that olive oil can help to lower blood pressure and improve the regulation of blood sugars as well as helping to reduce levels of cholesterol in the blood. Considering all these benefits, olive oil and peanut oil should become the main sources of oil in your diet. Approximately one-third of your total dietary fat intake will consist of monounsaturated fats on the Winning Weigh nutritional program.

Because of their high fat content, avocadoes, olives, and nuts are high in calories and will increase your total fat intake quickly. On the Winning Weigh diet system, you may eat avocadoes occasionally because they are high in vitamins. However, it is best to avoid nuts and olives altogether.

Conveniently, olive oil, peanut oil, and canola oil also contain small amounts of polyunsaturated fats. Your body does need some polyunsaturated fats, but not the excess found in corn oil and related polyunsaturated fat oils.

Exhibit 2–11
The Benefits of Olive Oil and Peanut Oil

- They help lower the level of cholesterol in your blood.
- They help lower your blood pressure.
- They improve the regulation of blood sugar.
- They are not as carcinogenic when exposed to light, heat, or oxygen as polyunsaturated vegetable oils are, and they do not make your blood sticky.
- They help maintain HDL levels (the good cholesterol).

So always use olive oil or peanut oil in place of polyunsaturated oils.

Omega 3 Fats

The fourth and final family of fats are the Omega 3 fats. Omega 3 fats are a special type of polyunsaturated fat found almost exclusively in fish and seafood. In general, the higher the fat content of the fish, the greater the amount of Omega 3 fats it has.

Exhibit 2–12
Fish and Seafood Especially High in Omega 3 Fats

> Anchovies, clams, crab, halibut, herring, mackerel, mullet, mussels, red snapper, rockfish, salmon, sardines, shad, swordfish, trout, tuna

Some populations, such as the Inuit and people in Japanese fishing villages, have especially low incidences of heart disease and cancer, so researchers studied these groups to see what they were doing right. Their findings suggest that people who rely substantially on fish (particularly fatty fish) as their main source of protein have significantly smaller risks of heart disease, related cardiovascular conditions, large bowel cancer, and cancers of the reproductive organs than the population at large. The Inuit who have migrated to Eastern Canada and the Japanese who have moved to North America have adopted our typical North American diet, high in saturated fats. As a result, their incidence of cardiovascular disease and cancer has become the same as ours.

Omega 3 fats seem to lower blood cholesterol levels significantly when they are substituted for foods high in saturated fats. Preliminary intervention studies have shown that when people with high levels of cholesterol in their blood eat more fatty fish, their cholesterol levels are reduced.

Omega 3 fats also make your blood less likely to form clots on the inside of your blood-vessel walls. These clots are often the first step in the development of hardening of the arteries. The clot acts like a glue that causes cholesterol to stick to that spot. As cholesterol builds up there, the blood vessel becomes even more narrow and plugged. Smoking cigarettes and eating a diet high in saturated and polyunsaturated fats are factors that increase the likelihood of abnormal blood clotting and thus create sites for blockages to occur.

Because of these benefits of Omega 3 fats, eating fatty fish is encouraged on the Winning Weigh program.

Fighting the Fat Temptation

Without a doubt, foods that are high in fat, especially saturated fat, are considered the most delicious and satisfying in our society. From our experience with our patients, we have found that the biggest dietary challenge for most people is cutting back on the amount of fat they eat. It is also the most important and life-enhancing change you can make in your diet. So it's up to you to start overcoming the fat temptations in your life.

We know that you're going to have some butter or mayonnaise or even ice cream from time to time. It's almost impossible not to. And it's not the end of the world either. It's what you generally do on ordinary days that really matters. The occasional slip-up is part of life. Just keep making wellness choices from moment to moment and with time you will have fewer and fewer setbacks. Don't feel that all is lost the first time you eat a food that is not on the Winning Weigh program.

Make a commitment to yourself *now* to cut back on the amount of fat you eat. Then, begin to make these promises a reality. See in your mind's eye that dietary fat is public health enemy number one. The ball is in your court. Take control of the game.

Starting Right Now . . .

1. When you eat high-fat foods, visualize the arterial plaque that is building up on the inside of your artery walls. This habit is the first step in overcoming the temptation to eat

high-fat, disease-promoting foods.
2. Stop using butter – it is almost pure saturated fat. Spread a little jam on toast. Moisten sandwiches with lettuce, tomato, cucumber, and a touch of olive oil as they do in Mediterranean countries.
3. Try hard to avoid all foods that are high in cholesterol and saturated fat. Switch to low-fat dairy products (skim milk, low-fat cheeses, "light" sour cream, and low-fat yogurt) and low-fat flesh products (poultry and fish).
4. Think twice before eating foods advertised as being "cholesterol-free." They may be high in saturated fat, which turns on your body's production of cholesterol. Especially avoid products that list palm, palm kernel, or coconut oil on the list of ingredients.
5. Use margarine and processed peanut butter only occasional-ly, if at all. They contain partially hydrogenated fats, which can elevate cholesterol levels and increase the stickiness of your blood.
6. Use olive oil or peanut oil instead of other vegetable oils for cooking and salads. Don't use corn oil, sunflower seed oil, soybean oil, safflower oil, or mixed vegetable oils in cooking. Exposure to heat can make them carcinogenic.
7. Avoid any kind of oil that has been exposed to high heat or left open to the air for a long time. Oil reused for deep-fat frying is usually loaded with free radicals, so avoid deep-fried foods, such as fish and chips.
8. Choose varieties of fish that are especially high in Omega 3 fats.
9. List some of the changes you intend to make in your eating habits on page 308 of your Wellness Planner.

Protein Foods and Their Nutrients

In our society, the major sources of dietary protein are foods of animal origin – meat, poultry, fish, and dairy products. As you have seen in the preceding chapter, some of these same foods are very high in saturated fat and cholesterol, substances you should avoid in a healthy diet. Therefore, the Winning Weigh program will direct you toward low-fat protein foods.

It's important for you to understand the purpose that protein serves in your diet. The principal role of dietary protein is to provide the major framework for your muscles, bones, teeth, hair, nails, and other body structures. It helps build and rebuild your body structure from day to day. As well, protein is used for other specialized roles such as enzyme formation, transportation of nutrients through the bloodstream, immune system functions, hormone formation, and more.

In the old days, many athletes ate a pregame steak, thinking that its protein provided energy for the upcoming event. But your body prefers to burn carbohydrates and fats for energy rather than protein. Research shows that athletes do better if they eat a meal that is rich in complex carbohydrates a few hours prior to the time when they will need their peak energy. Bread, pasta, rice, vegetable soups, fruit salads, baked potatoes, and bean salads are the pregame foods of choice today. They provide high-octane carbohydrate energy that enhances speed and endurance when combined with a proper training program.

However, consuming the right amount of protcin each day is critical to your health. Without any protein, you would die. But since adults primarily need protein only for replacement and since you don't lose much protein each day, you really don't need very much in your diet. Your body's genetic requirement is approximately 12 to 15 percent of your total calories each day (like fats and carbohydrates, protein is measured in calories even though it is not primarily used by your body as fuel).

Many people consume more protein food than they need. Too much protein intake forces the body to convert some of the excess protein to saturated fat. And that, of course, encourages heart disease, strokes, and cancer development in the reproductive organs. Additionally, a high protein intake generates by-products, such as urea and uric acid, that stress the kidneys and may encourage gouty arthritis in some people.

Many of the protein foods people eat also contain a lot of saturated fat and cholesterol. So the days of eating bacon and eggs for breakfast (protein and fat), ham and cheddar cheese sandwiches for lunch (protein and fat), and steak and French fries for dinner (protein and fat) ought to be put firmly in the past.

The kind of protein you eat is almost as important as the amount. The most common sources of protein are meat, dairy products, and some vegetables. While important health benefits can follow from an intelligent vegetarian diet, we know that most North Americans are not willing to stop eating meat. The Winning Weigh program will guide you toward low-fat protein foods of animal origin. If you want to make the commitment to adopt a strict vegetarian diet, consult other books. A vegetarian diet must be carefully planned and followed, so study the subject before you take that step.

We encourage you to eat two categories of low-fat protein foods each day. To make planning easy, have one meal containing low-fat flesh and one meal containing a low-fat dairy product. Both of these protein sources are important and contribute other unique properties to health promotion.

Protein from Low-Fat Dairy Foods

Once a day, you should eat a generous serving of a low-fat dairy product, such as low-fat milk, yogurt, or cheese. Knowing whether or not a dairy protein food meets the Winning Weigh requirement for low fat content is simple. Almost all dairy products display the percentage of milk fat (abbreviated "% M.F.") on the container. A low-fat cheese will contain 10% M.F. or less. A low-fat milk, buttermilk, or yogurt will contain 1% M.F. or less. If you restrict your dairy intake to these products, you will help ensure that your total calories from fat will be less than 25 percent. These foods are important not only because they are high in protein and low in cholesterol but because they contain essential minerals and vitamins, most notably calcium and vitamin D.

Exhibit 2–13
Low-Fat Dairy Products on the Winning Weigh

Skim or 1% milk
Yogurt (1% M.F. or less)
Cheese with 10% M.F. or less, for example,
- low-fat mozzarella
- ricotta
- cottage cheese
- farmer's cheese
- Neufchâtel
- sour cream (no more than 5 to 10% M.F.)
- buttermilk (skim or 1% M.F.)

Other low-fat products

Calcium from Low-Fat Dairy Foods

Calcium is essential to your health at all ages. As well as building strong bones and teeth, it prevents post-menopausal osteoporosis, a condition in which calcium is reabsorbed from the bones back into the bloodstream and then passed out of the body as urine, leaving the bones prone to fracture. Osteoporosis has been affecting more and more people in our society. In the United States alone it affects 15 to 20 million people and accounts for 1.3 million fractures each year. This condition mainly affects women due to the interaction between calcium and estrogen.

Estrogen, one of the female reproductive hormones, somehow helps the body retain calcium in bone. Production of the hormone is partially dependent on the size of fat cells. Fat cells can shrink to the point where they no longer produce enough estrogen to keep calcium in bone.

Many young women today are so obsessed with staying slim that they diet and exercise excessively. Their fat cells shrink to the point that they no longer produce the estrogen they need. Later in life, this condition will be worsened by the natural decrease in estrogen production after menopause.

In most cases, osteoporosis is almost completely preventable if your calcium intake is adequate throughout your lifetime, you remain physically active, and you maintain a healthy weight. You should also know that smoking and alcohol comsumption encourage osteoporosis.

The richest and most easily absorbed sources of calcium are dairy products. Numerous studies indicate that the calcium from dairy products is readily absorbed for use in the body for bone formation and a variety of other essential functions. The vitamin D in dairy products improves the absorption of calcium from the intestines to the bloodstream.

Osteoporosis is primarily a problem for women, but men also require calcium every day. Calcium is important for normal heart rhythm, muscle contractions, blood clotting, and the maintenance of normal blood pressure. Some preliminary evidence also suggests that optimal calcium intake can help reduce high blood pressure and prevent its onset. Calcium and vitamin D may also be important in the prevention of colon cancer. So adequate calcium is essential for both men and women at all ages.

Until women are about 35 years old, calcium from the bloodstream is delivered to bones to make them stronger. After that age, calcium no longer builds stronger bones, but it does slow down the rate at which calcium is absorbed from the bones back into the bloodstream. Your daily requirement of calcium increases with age, but 800 to 1000 mg per day is generally enough for both women and men. One eight-ounce serving of low-fat yogurt provides you with 350 to 400 mg of calcium. An eight-ounce glass of milk contains about 300 mg. As for cheeses, three or four ounces of most varieties will provide 300 to 400 mg of calcium. However, there are exceptions. Eight ounces of cottage cheese has only 140 mg of calcium. Ricotta cheese is very low in fat but also quite low in calcium, providing about half the amount of other cheeses. Because these two cheeses are lower in fat content and calories, you can choose generous servings of them to attain the desired amount of calcium. A balanced diet will also provide calcium through complex carbohydrate sources such as green leafy vegetables (spinach, collard greens, Swiss chard), beans, peas, kale, broccoli, bread, and grain products. Some women may require further calcium supplements. Every case is different, so you should see your physician if you are concerned.

Protein from Low-Fat Flesh Foods

Low-fat flesh provides the second source of protein on the Winning Weigh program. These foods are not only an important source of high-quality protein, but they are low in fat and cholesterol as well. They are also the major dietary source of two very important nutrients: vitamin B_{12} and iron. Both of these nutrients are essential for the normal production of red blood cells, which carry oxygen through the bloodstream. On the Winning Weigh program, you eat one serving per day of a low-fat flesh food.

**Exhibit 2–14
Low-Fat Flesh Foods on the Winning Weigh**

Chicken
Turkey
Cornish hens
Fish
Seafood

Vitamin B_{12}

Vitamin B_{12} is an essential ingredient for the normal reproduction and replication of all your body cells. Your cells need it in order to pass on precise genetic material from one generation of cells to the next. An inadequate intake of vitamin B_{12} is very serious, as cells can become unable to reproduce normally. The new generation of cells are large and abnormal looking, a condition known as ***megablastosis.*** They are unable to deliver oxygen to the tissues properly.

Cells with short life spans are the first to be affected by vitamin B_{12} deficiency. The cells that line the respiratory and intestinal tracts may be replaced after only 7 to 14 days. Red blood cells live only 120 days. Severe vitamin B_{12} deficiency also affects the nervous system.

Flesh foods are one of the only sources of vitamin B_{12}. Vegetarians are prone to vitamin B_{12} deficiency because most vegetables, grains, cereals, fruits, legumes, and dairy products do not contain appreciable amounts of vitamin B_{12}. The Winning Weigh program ensures that you receive sufficient amounts of vitamin B_{12} while still enjoying the benefits that a vegetarian diet would bring – low fat and cholesterol and a high concentration of complex carbohydrate foods.

Iron

Many people think of spinach and lentils as being high in iron, and in fact they are. However, the presence of fiber makes the iron in plant foods difficult to absorb from the intestine into the bloodstream. Fiber, which has a negative charge, attracts iron, which has a positive charge. The fiber drags up to 95 percent of the iron through the intestines, where it is ultimately expelled as part of the feces. So a large percentage of the iron from vegetables, cereals, and legumes is not used by your body at all.

The most easily digested and absorbed sources of iron are flesh foods. This iron, called ***heme*** iron, is bound to protein, so it is easily absorbed into the bloodstream. Chicken, turkey, Cornish hen, and most fish are all rich sources of dietary iron. They will enable you to maintain adequate stores of this important nutrient in your tissues.

As a component of hemoglobin in red blood cells, iron has the vital role of transporting oxygen – picking it up from the lungs and transporting it to every cell in your body. Iron is vital for energy production and immune system functioning. Iron deficiency is the number one mineral deficiency around the world. Up to 50 percent of women may have at least grade one iron deficiency because they don't get enough iron and they routinely lose blood through menstruation. Grade one deficiency leads to fatigue, weakness, and a depressed immune system. Later, more serious problems can develop, including the more extreme condition of iron deficiency anemia.

Eating one low-fat flesh food every day, combined with a variety of vegetables, cereals, beans, and peas, is a prudent strategy to get your daily iron requirement of approximately 18 mg per day. As with calcium, additional iron from a supplement may help help some people. The suggested range a supplement should provide is 10 to 18 mg of iron. Your physician will be able to determine early iron deficiency by assessing your serum ferratin levels.

Protein in Complex Carbohydrates

Your principal protein staples should include one low-fat dairy food and one low-fat flesh protein every day. These portions should provide for about 12 to 15 percent of your total calories every day. However, complex carbohydrate foods, which make up 55 to 65 percent of your daily food intake on the Winning Weigh, contain a supplemental amount of protein to ensure that you are getting adequate amounts every day. Most complex carbohydrates (except fruit) contain small but important amounts of protein. Especially good sources of protein are corn, potatoes, rice, pasta, peas, beans, and many breads and cereals. They provide the perfect complement to your daily flesh and dairy protein foods, providing protein without additional fat.

Starting Right Now . . .

1. Cut back on the amount of protein you eat. Eat only one serving of a low-fat dairy food and one serving of a low-fat flesh food every day.

2. Begin to collect recipes for preparing low-fat flesh and dairy foods such as chicken, fish, and low-fat cheese. Often you can adapt your favorite recipes by cutting back on the fat and making simple substitutions. Record some of your ideas on page 309 of your Wellness Planner. See Step 3 for ideas on preparing healthy meals and for a list of recommended wellness-oriented cookbooks.

Water and Other Fluids

The fifth nutritional component in your diet is water. Many people walk around every day in a semi-dehydrated state, **yet nearly every chemical reaction that takes place in your body requires water.** This is why severe dehydration can lead to death so quickly. All the essential life processes shut down when you are severely dehydrated.

To ensure that your body functions at an optimal level, you should drink six to eight glasses (1.5 to 2 quarts or litres) of water or other fluids every day. Maintaining enough water in your bloodstream is necessary for transporting essential nutrients to your tissues and for pushing your blood through the kidneys. Even partial dehydration will impair your kidneys' ability to filter toxins and waste products from your blood.

Water is also important for improving your metabolic efficiency and for burning fat in your tissue cells. If you don't drink enough water, losing weight will take longer.

Water also flushes excess sodium out of your body. Sodium is linked to high blood pressure in some people. Diuretic foods – foods that increase urine output – also help your body eliminate unwanted sodium. All fruits and vegetables in their natural states (not canned or processed) are diuretic foods. These natural diuretic foods can work only as long as you are getting enough water to drink each day.

Exhibit 2-15
Benefits of Drinking Enough Water

- Sufficient water keeps the pressure in your bloodstream high enough to transport nutrients to your tissues and to push your blood through your kidneys.

- It contributes to overall metabolic efficiency, including burning fat, making it easier to lose weight.

- It flushes excess sodium out of your body. Excess sodium also disturbs the balance of nutrients in your cells.

Salt (Sodium)

North Americans eat too much salt. Food manufacturers add sodium to everything we eat, from pickles to pancake mix. Most North Americans consume between 1600 and 2300 mg of sodium per day just from commercially processed foods. They get another 1200 mg from the sodium that occurs naturally in food. They consume a further 1300 to 2500 mg from the salt they add to food in the kitchen or at the dinner table. That brings the total average daily consumption of sodium to somewhere between 4100 and 6000 mg. Unfortunately, the U.S. Food and Nutrition Board recommends that healthy adults consume only 1100 to 3300 mg of sodium per day.

The Dangers of a High-Sodium Diet

The effect of excess sodium intake over a lifetime is strongly correlated with the development of high blood pressure. Approximately 9 to 20 percent of the population will get high blood pressure if their sodium intake is too high. High blood pressure has three side effects: strokes, heart attacks, and kidney failure.

Among the Kalahari bushmen of South Africa or the Melanesian tribes of New Guinea, sodium intake is low (200 to 1400 mg per day) and high blood pressure is virtually non-existent. In these primitive societies, unlike our own, blood pressure does not tend to increase with advancing age. However, when primitive societies adopt more modern ways of living, including increasing their intake of sodium, high blood pressure problems become much more prevalent. In northern Japan, the average sodium intake is astronomical – 9200 mg per day. Predictably, high blood pressure is a major problem.

In a study at the Mayo clinic, patients with high blood pressure reduced their intake of sodium to no more than 2000 mg each day. Patients with mild to moderate conditions of high blood pressure showed a significant reduction in blood pressure. (The results were not significant for patients with severe blood pressure.)

Many other clinical trials have supported these findings. It is increasingly apparent that excess sodium intake can spell trouble for some people.

Excess sodium can also lead to water retention and bloating. Because sodium binds water, it tends to interfere with the body's ability to properly regulate water balance.

As if all this is not enough reason for cutting back on your salt intake, excess sodium is mildly toxic and caustic to body tissues.

Cutting Back on Sodium

Our distant ancestors are partly to blame for our high sodium intake. They had a difficult time consuming enough sodium to sustain life. Over the generations, our bodies compensated by evolving a very elaborate hormonal system to prevent sodium from leaving the body. The kidneys work as sodium retainers. They filter undesirable components from the blood and into the urine, but they hold the sodium and return it to the bloodstream after filtering. Thus, your body does not get rid of excess sodium easily, and its negative effects tend to accumulate with time. The only effective strategy for avoiding the dangers of excess sodium is to drink plenty of water, eat plenty of diuretic foods, and decrease your intake of sodium.

Even though prepared foods and fast foods already contain a lot of sodium, one-fourth to one-third of your daily sodium intake is discretionary. You can control whether or not you eat it. If you cut down or eliminate the salt you add to food and cut back on high-sodium processed foods and beverages, you can keep your sodium intake within safe boundaries.

Because you are accustomed to a lot of sodium in your food, you may find that unsalted foods taste a little flat. Don't worry; soon the nerve endings on your tongue will begin to transmit new and interesting tastes to your brain and the real flavors of the food will begin to emerge. Your taste buds will reawaken and, eventually, you'll find you no longer like salty foods.

If you find it difficult to give up the taste of salt on your food, you might use a salt substitute instead. Most of these contain

Exhibit 2–16
Some Sodium Facts

Table salt (sodium chloride) is 40 percent sodium by weight. One teaspoon of salt contains 2000 mg of sodium.

One cup of canned or packaged soup usually contains approximately 900 mg of sodium.
One dill pickle contains about 1000 mg of sodium.

Baking soda, baking powder, meat sauces, gravies, and mixes are loaded with sodium. So is MSG (monosodium glutamate), a flavor enhancer found in many Chinese foods.

Prepared condiments, including relish, catsup, pickles, mustard, soya sauce, Worcestershire sauce, and olives are often very high in sodium.

Most soft drinks, such as diet cola and soda water, contain less than 20 mg of sodium per cup.

Sodium chloride, sodium saccharin, sodium benzoate, sodium nitrate, and sodium nitrite are all common sodium additives. Read labels carefully to watch for sodium levels.

All fresh fruits and vegetables contain more potassium than sodium. Because it is a diuretic, potassium helps the body excrete excess sodium.

potassium in place of sodium. If you suffer from any form of kidney trouble, check with your doctor to make sure that additional potassium will not harm you.

Exhibit 2–17
Foods that contain . . .

less than 25 mg of sodium
12 oz. soda water
12 oz. diet soft drinks

less than 75 mg of sodium
3 oz. chicken
3 oz. turkey
3 oz. fresh fish
3 oz. canned tuna or salmon (low-sodium, water-packed)

less than 120 mg of sodium
1 cup low-fat milk
1 cup low-fat yogurt
1/2 cup cottage cheese
1/4 cup shellfish
3 oz. shrimp
3/4 cup lobster
3/4 cup oysters
2 oz. clams
1 slice bread
3 low-fat crackers

less than 240 mg of sodium
1 oz. of most low-fat cheeses
1/2 cup of tomato juice
2 tbsps. of prepared Italian dressing
1 cup of most breakfast cereals

less than 360 mg of sodium
1 oz. turkey or chicken breast cold cuts
5 olives

less than 1000 mg of sodium
2 tsp. baking powder
1 bouillon cube
1 dill pickle
1/2 tsp. table salt
1 cup of canned or packaged soups

Sources of Fluids

Water

Water should be your most important source of fluids. Unfortunately, tap water is always an unknown quantity. You never really know how safe it is. The United States Environmental Protection Agency (EPA) has found over 700 organic chemicals in drinking water. Forty of these chemicals have been shown to cause cancer in laboratory animals. Three of these chemicals – benzene, chloromethyl ether, and vinyl chloride – are associated with cancer in humans.

The standards for water quality in the United States established by the EPA allow municipalities to average their water's impurities over a year. Those averages are likely to look far more reassuring than the extremes. In summer, for instance, much more chlorine is added to water to control microorganisms than would be used for the rest of the year. Some cities exceed EPA standards for chlorine by 20 percent during mid-summer. Nitrates and pesticides are also likely to be found in drinking water during the summer; both of those also carry the threat of cancer development. A number of studies demonstrate that contaminated water has been associated with an increased risk of cancer and other medical problems. Drinking polluted water has been identified by the EPA as one of the top for health hazards threatening Americans.

Make sure that your drinking water is safe. Having a high-quality water purification system attached to your home plumbing is often a smart idea. Have your water tested by a laboratory if you have any doubts about its purity. If you use bottled water, select brands that have undergone distillation, reverse osmosis, or a combination of reverse osmosis and deionization.

Coffee and Tea

Caffeine in large quantities (40 cups or more of coffee per week) has been linked to cancer of the pancreas and the bladder. It seems to inhibit your cells from correcting genetic mistakes. However, the evidence overwhelmingly indicates that having two cups of coffee or tea per day is not a risk factor for any terrible diseases. Have it black: the fat in cream, milk, and non-dairy creamer is not good for you. Neither is sugar. If you are trying to cut down on caffeine, try drinking water-treated decaffeinated coffee or, even better, hot water with lemon, herbal teas, or coffee substitutes.

Alcohol

Studies show that one to two alcoholic drinks per day may actually reduce your risk of heart disease. (One drink equals one beer, a five-ounce glass of wine, or one ounce of hard liquor.) This effect is probably due to its influence in raising HDL cholesterol (the good cholesterol) levels. However, aerobic exercise is a better way to raise your HDL levels.

Alcohol is loaded with empty calories and is a known co-carcinogen, in that it carries free radicals into the cells, allowing them to cause genetic damage. For example, smoking cigarettes contributes to cancers of the lungs, mouth, esophagus, stomach, bladder, pancreas, and kidney. However, if you smoke and drink at the same time, alcohol acts as a co-carcinogen and your risk of getting mouth cancer increases 15 times compared to smoking without drinking. Alcohol speeds up the delivery of free radicals to your genetic material. It also carries many impurities into the body that may indirectly increase your risk of cancer.

In the long run, you will probably be more healthy if you don't drink alcohol. If you do drink, we recommend that you limit yourself to one or two drinks in any one day.

Juice

When you drink juice, dilute it first. Drink 1/4 cup of unsweetened juice with 3/4 cup of water. Pure juice has had much of the fiber stripped away, so the sugar in the juice, whether added or natural, is digested too fast, resulting in a bombardment of glucose into your bloodstream.

Diet Soft Drinks and Soda Water

Most soft drinks also cause a sugar rush that produces the various undesirable reactions in your body that we described in the section on white sugar. If you particularly like the taste of soft drinks, no one has yet proven that one drink of a diet soft drink each day is likely to do you any harm; however, we feel that soda water with lemon or lime would be a wiser choice.

Exhibit 2-18
Sources of Fluids on the Winning Weigh Program

Drink six to eight glasses (1.5 to 2 quarts or litres) of fluids every day. We recommend

water that has undergone reverse osmosis (and perhaps deionization)

distilled water

pure spring water from deep sources below the ground

low-sodium mineral water

low-sodium soda water

1 part unsweetened juice diluted with 3 parts water

skim or 1% milk

Starting Right Now . . .

Pay attention to how much you are drinking now. Increase this by one or two glasses a week until you work up to six to eight glasses of fluids each day. (By the way, coffee, tea, and alcohol don't count as fluids because their fluid content is offset by the fact that they increase water loss through urination.)

Exercise

The human body has over 600 muscles, giving it a tremendous capacity for movement and physical activity. Regular physical activity is as much a natural way of living as breathing in oxygen. Yet the average North American moves very little. Our activity level has been reduced by cars, washing machines, assembly lines, farm equipment, supermarkets, elevators, snow blowers, and golf carts, to name only a few movement-saving devices.

Going against our genetic blueprints in this way leads inevitably to disease and degeneration. The progressive decline in physical activity during this century has paralleled and contributed to the rise in obesity, heart disease, and cancer.

We have to find twentieth century substitutes for the activities we no longer need to perform. Walking, jogging, cycling, rowing, swimming, aerobics, dancing: there are lots of alternatives. Your body demands a minimum amount of physical activity every week. If it doesn't get enough, it undergoes a degenerative process that can be likened to starvation.

Even if your diet is ideal, your muscles will degenerate and shrink without adequate exercise. They will also become more susceptible to tears and ruptures. They will no longer adequately support your joints, especially your hips, knees, and lower back. You will be prone to osteoarthritis. Your bones will lose calcium more easily, increasing your chance of developing osteoporosis. Without adequate physical activity, you can count on progressive deterioration of your muscle and bone structure, your cardiovascular integrity, your digestive tract, and your other organ systems.

Exercise is one of the most empowering activities there is. You commit yourself, you carry out your intentions, and you enjoy the benefits. Many of the people we counsel have begun with a simple exercise program three times a week. Then they used the enthusiasm, self-confidence, and organization skills they gained to enrich their lives with other activities that contributed to their personal growth activities.

The Importance of Aerobic Exercise

Aerobic exercise increases the participant's oxygen intake and heart rate. Regular participation in an aerobic exercise program prevents the deterioration of your body, as well as bringing a huge number of positive health benefits. By aerobic exercise, we mean any activity that accelerates your heart rate within what is known as the "aerobic training zone" for a minimum of 20 minutes (ideally 30 to 60 minutes) at least three times a week. You should exercise at a level of intensity that has you breathing harder than normal but that still allows you to carry on a conversation. Examples of aerobic exercise include jogging, stationary cycling, rowing, long-distance swimming, cross-country skiing, and dancing. All of these forms of exercise provide many health benefits.

Cardiovascular Benefits

Aerobic exercise improves the capacity of your body tissues to extract oxygen from red blood cells, transport it to the inside of the cells, and use it for energy production. Although your red blood cells are always saturated with more oxygen than your body requires at any given moment, the ability of the tissues to pick up this oxygen can vary greatly from one person to the next. An aerobically fit person picks up oxygen from the bloodstream about 25 percent more efficiently than someone who is unfit. And the more oxygen your tissues can pick up, the less stressful it is for your heart to deliver adequate quantities of oxygen to your tissues.

Light activity alone does not significantly improve the utilization of oxygen in your body. You must maintain an increased heart rate for at least 20 minutes three times a week to create these aerobic adaptations. In just six to eight weeks, the average person can increase his or her oxygen consumption by 10 to 15 percent through aerobic exercise.

The benefits of improved oxygen utilization are enormous. You will have more energy. Your tissues will become more efficient at using the oxygen that is already there so your heart will be under less stress. Your heart will also become stronger and able to pump more blood through your body with every beat. Thus, it can beat more slowly and still provide adequate blood to your body. On average, an aerobically fit person actually has a slower resting heart rate (48 to 66 beats per minute) than an aerobically unfit person (72 to 99 beats per minute).

A slower resting heart beat is a tremendous advantage in itself. Between heart beats, your heart can deliver blood to its own coronary vessels and supply itself with more oxygen. To appreciate the importance of these aerobic adaptations, keep in mind that a heart attack occurs when your heart muscle cannot get the oxygen it needs. So the better equipped your heart is to deliver oxygen to its own muscles, the better off you are.

But that's not all. Studies also show that aerobically fit exercisers have higher levels of HDL cholesterol ("good" cholesterol) in their bloodstream. HDL cholesterol helps to prevent the arteries from narrowing and may even reverse the narrowing process.

Stress Reduction

Aerobic exercise lowers psychological stress by balancing and regulating hormones that promote high blood pressure. During periods of stress, the amount of adrenaline hormone in your system increases. During aerobic exercise, your body releases adrenaline slowly and regularly; after exercising, your level of adrenaline returns to the ideal baseline. Thus, aerobic exercise can help you relieve stress and retard the development of high blood pressure.

Many highly stressed people have discovered that aerobic exercise helps them unwind. It's also a great way to clear the cobwebs from your head and reduce the mental pressures of the day. In fact, aerobic exercise takes you into an "altered" state of consciousness that triggers positive thoughts, making it a powerful mind-body experience. For example, it is well-documented that exercise helps prevent recurring depression. It induces **runner's high,** the heightened mood state that usually kicks in 20 to 30 minutes into an aerobic workout session. Some research indicates that this high is actually created by the release of pleasure-giving brain chemicals know as endorphins.

Finally, exercise affects your appetite and food choices. Most people find it easier to make healthy food choices after an exercise routine. The appetite center seems to prefer healthier, lighter foods.

Fat Reduction

Losing a few extra pounds can also help lower your blood pressure and reduce your risk of cardiovascular disease. Two-thirds of overweight people with high blood pressure could bring their blood pressure down to normal simply by losing some of their excess weight. Losing excess weight also helps lower elevated levels of triglycerides (fats) in the blood. Triglycerides are linked to heart disease and related cardiovascular conditions.

You can be trim and slender but still unfit from an aerobic point of view. Conversely, you can be in great aerobic shape even if you are overweight. No matter how much you weigh, you can attain great benefits to your heart, cardiovascular system, and muscle tissues from aerobic exercise. Being aerobically fit actually helps minimize some of the risks of being overweight. So don't wait to lose weight before you begin an aerobic exercise program.

Spot-reducing exercises such as sit-ups and leg lifts will tone the muscles under the fat, but they will not eliminate fat itself. Only aerobic exercise can stimulate the release of fat from your fat cells. Here's how it works. Let's say you get on a stationary bicycle and begin peddling. As your heart beat speeds up, your nervous system releases adrenaline. Adrenaline triggers the breakdown of fat in your fat cells everywhere in your body, not just in the muscles you are exercising. Individual fat molecules escape from your fat cells and enter the bloodstream, where they circulate through your body. The exercising muscles (including the heart and respiratory muscles) pick up the circulating fat molecules and burn them to generate energy. The longer the aerobic exercise continues, the more fat is released and burned.

After the Exercise Stops

For a long time after you stop exercising, your muscles continue to pick up and burn the fat already in your bloodstream. However, your tissues will stop releasing fat molecules into your bloodstream very rapidly because your demand for energy decreases.

Several factors affect how long you burn fat after exercise. Most significantly, the longer the exercise session, the more fat will be released from your fat cells and therefore the more fat is burned after exercise. Ideally, you should build up until you are doing a 45-minute workout at each session. A 45-minute session also significantly depletes the carbohydrate stores in your muscles and liver. Your body will be so busy rebuilding these stores that most of your tissue cells will continue to burn fat as their primary fuel even when you are at rest. (If you are following the Winning Weigh nutrition program, which is rich in carbohydrates, you will not experience the symptoms of low blood sugar, or hypoglycemia.)

Resisted weight training exercises (such as bench press, Nautilus®, barbell, and dumbbell exercises) encourage fat breakdown after aerobic exercise is over because they tremendously deplete your muscles' carbohydrate stores. While your body is rebuilding its stores, your cells continue to burn fat. Weight training also has other benefits, including increasing your strength, improving your posture, and helping to prevent the weakening of your musculoskeletal system. If you do not maintain the strength and flexibility of your muscles, you can more easily develop sprains, strains, and wear-and-tear damage over your lifetime.

Also, muscles are more metabolically active than fat tissues so they consume large amounts of energy even when they are resting. Therefore, the more muscular you are, the more calories you will burn at rest. You will have a faster metabolic rate.

If you are just beginning an aerobic exercise program, then you probably won't want to start with resisted weight training right away. However, when you become more experienced and more fit, ask a fitness instructor at a local health club to draw you up a starter program. With all the new sophisticated equipment available, resistance training can be safe for almost everyone.

Despite the many ways in which aerobic exercise helps you burn fat, you must realize that no exercise program alone can reverse the dangerous impact of a high-fat diet. A healthy diet and a good aerobic exercise program must work together for wellness.

The Benefits of Light Exercise

Does the thought of aerobic exercise go against every instinct in your body? Do you view exercise as unnecessary work that produces discomfort and fatigue? Despite the phenomenal growth of the wellness movement throughout the 1980s, many people are still vehemently opposed to doing strenuous exercise.

You can attain some of the benefits of regular exercise through a program of light activity, such as walking. Several recent studies have shown that burning 2000 calories per week in light physical activity increases longevity. For example, it lowers the risk of coronary heart disease by 39 percent and significantly lowers the risk of several other degenerative conditions, even if you are an overweight smoker with a history of high blood pressure. One source of evidence for this claim was provided in a famous study of Harvard alumni done by Dr. Paffenbarger. *A minimum amount of physical activity is an essential part of a wellness lifestyle.* And we're not talking about sweat and exertion here – 2000 calories' worth of walking will do it. For most people that would require a walk of 45 to 60 minutes (3 to 4 miles, or 5 to 6.5 km) four to six times per week.

Other research has been published showing that physical activity helps prevent colon cancer. It has also been linked with decreases in breast cancer. Exercise seems to regulate estrogren levels. During a woman's teenage years, excess body fat can establish a pattern of estrogen secretion that may hasten the onset of cancers in the reproductive tissues later in life. When fat cells increase in size because you have been overeating and not getting enough exercise, they may become overstimulated and increase the production of potentially harmful forms of estrogen.

This estrogen makes reproductive tissues more susceptible to cancer. According to research done by Rose Frisch, women who have a lifetime of exercise have a dramatically lower rate of reproductive organ cancers than women who have a history of little exercise.

Any way you look at it, the message is becoming quite clear. Physical activity does not need to be excessively demanding for it to be of value in the prevention of heart disease and cancer.

Exhibit 2–19
The Benefits of Exercise

Light Activity:
- lowers the risk of cardiovascular disease
- helps prevent cancer of the colon and rectum
- helps prevent breast cancer
- prevents the degeneration and shrinking of your muscles

Aerobic Exercise:
- provides all the benefits of light activity
- improves your body's ability to use oxygen from the bloodstream, thus making you more energetic and reducing strain on your heart
- slows down your resting heart beat so your heart has more time to deliver blood and oxygen to its own coronary vessels between beats
- increases the amount of HDL ("good") cholesterol in your bloodstream
- regulates and lowers your levels of stress-producing hormones, which contribute to high blood pressure
- helps prevent and dispel depression
- helps you feel good and helps you unwind
- makes you feel like eating healthier foods

- stimulates the release of fat molecules from your fat cells
- burns the fat molecules released from your cells even after you have finished exercising
- helps you lose weight, thus lowering your blood pressure and reducing your risk of cardiovascular disease

Starting Right Now . . .

1. Try to be more active. Walk up the stairs instead of using the elevator. Walk to the store instead of driving. Take a stroll just for fun.

2. Start thinking about what kind of regular exercise you would like to do.

3. Consider starting resisted weight training exercises to build-up muscle mass if you are already reasonably fit.

4. We know from our experience with patients over the years that the more real the benefits the Winning Weigh program provides for you, the better your chances for long-term success. You are following the Winning Weigh program because of the benefits it has to offer. So in order to make wellness a reality, you must focus on the benefits, both physical and psychological. Flip to the Wellness Planner (pp. 310-311) and rate how you feel about each of the benefits that you can achieve on the Winning Weigh program.

STEP 3   DISCOVERING THE FORMULA

The Winning Weigh Program

If you have read Step 2 carefully, you are now familiar with the essential ingredients of a health-promoting diet. The challenge that now faces you is to incorporate those nutritional principles into your daily eating habits. The Winning Weigh program provides a practical, easy-to-follow formula, which allows you to put your nutritional knowledge into action. Based on the general recommendations for good health published by the Heart and Stroke Foundation, the Cancer Society, and the Diabetes Association, this simple system will ensure that you get the combination of nutrients you need to reach your optimal level of health.

Once you incorporate the principles of the Winning Weigh program, remaining on track with your wellness goals will be easy. The Winning Weigh program can become your lifelong plan for healthy eating because it is the easiest wellness-oriented formula that you will ever encounter. By following this practical nutritional and lifestyle program, you will be defending yourself against heart disease, strokes, and cancers of the large intestine and reproductive organs. You will also improve your performance in both endurance and all-out-effort sports. In fact, the energy you gain on the Winning Weigh program will help you to improve in all aspects of your life.

As well as maintaining your high energy levels through a continuous supply of carbohydrates in your bloodstream, the Winning Weigh formula will also provide the other dietary building blocks: fiber, protein, fat, and water. In addition, the program will introduce you to a large variety of foods containing anti-cancer nutrients.

Finally, the program will help you to shed those extra pounds and keep them off without a continuous struggle. Say good-bye to fad diets, calorie counting, weight-loss clinics, hormone injection treatments, and all the other nonsense that leaves you weak, vulnerable, and desperate, not to mention broke.

If you want to **gain** weight, the regular Winning Weigh program can help you reach your goal if you combine it with a resistance weight training program.

For those of you who are used to reading diet books or following rigid plans, our approach to this step will be a new experience for you.

The Winning Weigh program can help you in various ways because it provides basic nutritional information and encourages you to use it to achieve your own goals.

Instead of specific recipes that you are to follow each day, *The Winning Weigh* offers you the recipe for wellness. After reading this section, you will have the power to judge any recipe on its health-promoting value. In addition, you will be able to adapt it to your needs and wants. Read Step 3 several times. Learn a foundation of facts so that they will spring to mind as you are reading recipes or menus or walking down the aisles of supermarkets. Reading ingredients of canned foods, packaged dry foods or prepared meals, you will begin to see where they fit into the Winning Weigh formula. In a restaurant, you will not just read the menu, but evaluate it and make substitutions that are in keeping with your health.

As much as we all wish for a formula that we can follow for the rest of our lives, there is an opposite force that wants to be strong and make independent choices. The two-staple system will begin to create a flexible structure for your lifetime of daily choices. It allows you to balance these two natural inclinations of human nature.

The Two Staples of the Winning Weigh Program

You really only need to be aware of two food staples on the Winning Weigh program, protein foods and complex carbohydrate foods.

Protein foods provide the building blocks of your body's structure: its muscles, bone, skin, hair, and nails. They are vital for the optimal performance of your immune system and the manufacture of specialized body proteins. One low-fat dairy and one low-fat flesh protein food per day will provide you with most of the protein you need. You will also get the bulk of your calcium, vitamin D, iron, and vitamin B$_{12}$ requirements from your daily protein foods.

Complex carbohydrate foods, those high-octane, high-energy foods, are converted by your body into glucose that powers every cell in your body. As you have read in Step 2, complex carbohydrate foods can also help you lose weight and many are high in dietary fiber and anti-cancer nutrients, making their nutritional contribution of vital importance.

On the Winning Weigh program, you do not have to keep track of a lot of food groups or numerous nutritional elements. Just make sure that every day you eat a flesh protein food, a dairy protein food, and a variety of complex carbohydrate foods. We will show you how to co-ordinate these elements into some simple meal plans.

Except for your fat intake, we don't regulate the portion sizes on this program. You should eat the amount of food that your body tells you it needs. Athletes, for example, may require twice as many daily calories as less active people. On the other hand, it is critically important that you don't overeat. Only you know how fast or slow your metabolism is and how much food you can eat without gaining weight. Because we don't know you personally, we can't tell you the exact quantities of food that are right for you. However, we do know what style of eating will promote your health and help prevent heart disease. Your job is to pay attention to your body's responses so you can determine the amount of food you need.

As we said earlier, the problem with going on someone else's diet is that it is someone else's diet. The Winning Weigh program is your program. You are in charge of choosing the right quantities of food for yourself. Because the Winning Weigh program limits your consumption of fat, you will probably find you can eat much more than you expected without gaining weight.

Exhibit 3–1
Protein Foods

Flesh Protein
chicken (skin removed)
turkey (skin removed)
Cornish game hens
fish
seafood
lean veal or beef (twice a month maximum)

Dairy Protein
low-fat cheese (less than 10% M.F.)
plain yogurt (less than 1% M.F.)
skim milk (less than 1% M.F.)

Complex Carbohydrates

fruit	vegetables
grains	bread products
pasta	cereals
jam	legumes (peas and beans)
clear soups	

The Winning Weigh Meal Plan

On the Winning Weigh program, you eat three different types of meals each day. Each type of meal includes a different combination of protein and complex carbohydrate foods, giving your genetic blueprint what it needs to provide good health and weight control. You may also eat between-meal snacks.

Exhibit 3–2
The Winning Weigh Meal Plan

1. Flesh-Protein Meal
- one low-fat flesh protein food
- two or more complex carbohydrate foods

2. Dairy-Protein Meal
- one low-fat dairy protein food
- two or more complex carbohydrate foods

3. Complex-Carbohydrate-Only Meal
- two or more complex carbohydrate foods

4. Between Meals (optional):
- complex carbohydrate snacks

You can have these three meals in any order. Your body operates on a 24-hour cycle, known as ***circadian rhythm.*** As long you have dairy protein, flesh protein, and complex-carbohydrate-only meals sometime during the day, you will experience the full benefits of the Winning Weigh program. For instance, one day you may have your dairy-protein meal for breakfast as yogurt and fruit. The next day, you may have it for dinner as cheese and spinach lasagna. All that matters is that you have one, and only one, dairy-protein meal every day.

Eating small snacks between meals is not necessarily a bad thing. It can help regulate your blood sugar, preventing you from getting tired and irritable. It can also prevent you from feeling deprived. Remember to eat only complex carbohydrate foods as snacks. A piece of fruit, melba toast with salsa, and unbuttered popcorn are great examples.

Notice that every meal on the Winning Weigh program includes complex carbohydrate foods. Eat a variety of these foods in order to get a wide range of nutrients. Pay special attention to complex carbohydrate foods that are rich in anti-cancer nutrients or high in fiber, such as whole wheat bread and breakfast cereals, orange and yellow fruits and vegetables, broccoli, cauliflower, and Brussels sprouts.

The Vegetarian Option

If, for any reasons, you want a vegetarian alternative to dairy and/or meat products, the Winning Weigh program offers you this flexibility. You will need to be sure, however, that you still get the protein, vitamins, and minerals you need. Before you eliminate dairy and/or flesh foods from your diet altogether, learn as much as you can about how to get the nutrients you need.

If you want to skip the flesh-protein meal, you must be sure to substitute it with a meal high in protein, vitamin B_{12}, and iron. Most soybean products are high in protein, but you should eat them with grain products such as rice, bread, or pasta. Tofu, miso, tempeh, and texturized vegetable proteins are all very high in protein. Beans and peas also provide large amounts of protein, but, like the soybean products, they should be eaten with grains. If you are using a vegetarian alternative on a long-term basis, you should also take a multiple vitamin and mineral supplement that includes the recommended daily allowance of vitamin B_{12} and iron.

If you want an alternative to the dairy-protein meal, you must be sure that you eat foods containing both protein and calcium. Some soybean products, such as tofu, are high in calcium and protein (when eaten with grain products). In addition to taking a multiple vitamin and mineral supplement, you should also consider taking a 600 to 800 mg calcium supplement every day.

Other Elements of the Winning Weigh Program

As well as making sure you have one dairy-protein meal, one flesh-protein meal, and one complex-carbohydrate-only meal every day, you must keep track of four other things to ensure that your diet is as healthy as possible – oil, water, cancer-preventing nutrients, and fiber. This tracking is amazingly easy once you get started.

Oils

You should add one to two teaspoons of monounsaturated oil to your diet every day to help keep your cholesterol level down. You could mix olive oil with vinegar to make salad dressings or sauté your vegetables in peanut oil. You may use a little margarine occasionally, but we don't recommend it for regular use. It is very important, however, *that you do not have more than two servings of these oils per day* – any more than that will increase your risk of cancer.

The remaining 20 to 25 percent of your total calories that come from fat should be from low-fat protein staples and, to a lesser degree, complex carbohydrate staples.

Water

Try to drink at least six to eight glasses of fluids every day. If possible, drink distilled water or water that has undergone a process of reverse osmosis and deionization. You can drink some soda water, mineral water, or water from a deep spring.

Fiber

To be healthy, you must satisfy your body's requirements for dietary fiber. As you read in Step 2, you should include two different kinds of fiber in your daily diet: cholesterol crunchers and colon cleaners. Cholesterol crunchers help keep your blood cholesterol levels low, and colon cleaners dilute the effects of cancer-causing agents that may be present in the colon and rectum.

It is often difficult to know whether you are eating enough fiber. The Winning Weigh Fiber Scoreboard (starting on p. 293) is your answer to this problem. Using the work of two prominent researchers, Southgate and Andersone, we have reviewed the fiber content of the most common foods containing cholesterol crunchers or colon cleaners. Each food has been given a point value, or *score.* One medium apple, for example, scores one fiber point, while half a cup of kidney beans scores three points.

On the Winning Weigh program, you should attain *8 to 15 fiber points every day.* This amount is based on the guidelines set out by the Cancer Society and the Heart and Stroke Foundation.

These 8 to 15 fiber points constitute your daily prescription for keeping your cholesterol level down, your glucose and insulin levels regulated, and your intestinal tract functioning properly.

You can get these fiber points every day by choosing fiber-rich complex carbohydrate foods and by supplementing your fiber intake with the Winning Weigh Fiber Mixture. Sprinkle it over your breakfast cereal or stir it into some yogurt with fresh fruit.

Exhibit 3-3
The Winning Weigh Fiber Mixture

one part oat bran
one part wheat bran or high-fiber wheat bran cereal

Mix up a large batch and use it every day.
Add some wheat germ to your daily serving.

To determine the number of fiber points a particular food has, look it up in the Fiber Scoreboard. You will very quickly learn which are the high-fiber foods. At the end of the day, simply add up your fiber points to see how you did.

Keeping on the Winning Weigh

Keep track of your progress on the Winning Weigh program. "Record makers are record breakers" is a motto worth remembering. Every day, write down everything you eat in a Daily Food, Fiber, and Activity Journal (see p. 323). You will find it much harder to cheat by sneaking small bites of foods that are high in saturated fats, for example, when you have to face your transgression in black and white. Recording your daily activities in a journal will give you a sense of power and control over this program and will help you stay on course.

Starting Right Now . . .

1. Make copies of the forms provided on pages 324-325 to create your Daily Food, Fiber, and Activity Journal. List all the foods you have eaten so far today. Calculate how many fiber points you have. Continue to list all the foods you eat, keeping track of your daily fiber intake using the Fiber Scoreboard (starting on page 293).

2. Start following the Winning Weigh program today! Here are some daily goals to set for yourself:

    a. Eat one low-fat dairy protein meal, one low-fat flesh protein meal, and one carbohydrate-only meal. All snacks should consist of complex carbohydrates only.

    b. Eat one to two teaspoons of monounsaturated oil (peanut or olive oil), but ***no more added fats.*** You can use these oils to make salad dressings or stir fried vegetables.

    c. Drink six to eight glasses of water or other allowable fluids.

    d. Eat foods containing 8 to 15 fiber points.

Making the Program Work

You now know that the Winning Weigh program offers you an approach to healthy eating. But you also know that there will be times when you will be faced with temptation. To help you develop a realistic way of gauging your performance, we have put together the Winning Weigh Food Chart (Exhibit 3-4). At the top of the chart, you will find the Wellness Foods that are recommended for the Winning Weigh program. If you consistently eat foods from this category and follow the Winning Weigh formula, you can rest assured that you will reach your nutritional goals for wellness.

There are foods, however, that are nutritious yet a little higher in fat than is desirable for everyday consumption. We have listed them in a second category called Compromise Foods. You can occasionally eat foods from this category without having to worry too much about getting off track. A bran muffin purchased from a doughnut shop, for instance, is too high in saturated fat to be considered a true wellness food. However, it is also a good source of complex carbohydrates and colon cleaner fiber. And it is certainly much better for you than a doughnut! So have a store-bought bran muffin once in a while, just not every day. The key thing is to keep moving forward. If you are accustomed to eating a bran muffin every day, try to cut that down to three times a week, then maybe twice a week. Gradually begin making more selections from the Wellness Foods category.

The third category consists of Recreational Foods. These foods should be viewed as treats, items you should not have more than once a week. They have minimal nutritional value but can sometimes help you get through those moments of weakness.

The fourth category, Hazardous Foods, speaks for itself. Try to avoid foods from this category. Remember, you are on the road to good health. Don't get sidetracked! If you feel tempted to eat hazardous foods, try eating something listed in the Compromise Foods or Recreational Foods first. You will probably find that your cravings disappear and that the temptation vanishes.

Exhibit 3–4
The Winning Weigh Food Chart

1. Wellness Foods – Right on track

all fruits	chicken and turkey
all vegetables	egg whites
cereal products	Cornish hens
grain products	fish and shellfish
peas and beans	low-fat milk
clear broth soups	low-fat yogurt
whole-fruit jam	low-fat cheese

2. Compromise Foods – The edge of wellness

muffins	pizza (1/2 the normal cheese)
humus with tahini	black coffee
2% milk products	soft-boiled or poached eggs
Caesar salad	chicken wings (baked, not fried)
(no bacon or cheese)	English muffins
chicken with skin	cheese (10% M.F. or less)
margarine (on bread or potatoes)	

3. Recreational Foods – Occasional treats

cappuccino	sherbet
fruit yogurt	frozen fruit ices
jujubes	licorice
pancakes	angel food cake
1 - 2 alcoholic beverages	

4. Hazardous Foods – Look for a less harmful substitute

red meat	high-fat salad dressings
luncheon meats	sausages
bacon	mayonnaise
cheese cake	high-fat pastries
whole milk	butter
fried eggs	omelets
spare ribs	pizza with a lot of cheese and pepperoni
doughnuts	ice cream
cream	cheese (over 10% M.F.)
waffles	

Using Substitutions to Make the Wish Come True

The Winning Weigh formula represents a goal that you're working toward, and you may never quite follow all our advice. Don't worry; there is room for flexibility. We are talking about a lifelong program, so we don't expect everyone to be perfect every moment. This is not an all-or-nothing process, but a gradual development of a wellness-oriented lifestyle.

Let's be realistic for a moment. Everyone begins the Winning Weigh program with some weaknesses: bacon and eggs on Sunday morning; cheddar cheese melting over a plate of nacho chips after a baseball game; potato chips and sour cream dip in front of the television; spare ribs; hamburgers and fries; cheesecake; banana splits...the list is endless. These disease-promoting habits are not something that you can just wish away. They are small addictions that you must overcome if you want to reduce your risk of serious disease.

Changing habits takes time. Be prepared for the occasional setback. You may stumble sometimes on the road to success, but don't be too hard on yourself. Just keep trying to change the hazardous behavior to patterns that are not quite so damaging.

Mrs. L. sold real estate. On her travels around town, Mrs. L. was in the habit of stopping at coffee-and-doughnut shops. Trying to cut down on her daily fat intake, she always intended to limit herself to coffee, which she drank black. Quite often, however, the aroma of the freshly baked doughnuts would tempt her to buy a treat along with her coffee. She knew she would hate herself if she did, yet two or three times a day she found herself caught up in the same pattern.

After working with her for several weeks, we helped her solve the dilemma. Instead of a doughnut, she would choose a bran muffin. To keep the calories down, she would only eat the top half of the muffin. That was her favorite part anyway! With this one simple substitution, Mrs. L. managed to completely cut doughnuts out of her daily routine.

Let's look at what happened. Once inside a doughnut shop, Mrs. L.'s desire for a doughnut was activated by the aroma. This urge overwhelmed her and she couldn't just walk away. But she was not totally powerless. She learned to step back and make a less damaging choice that still satisfied her craving. It would be better, of course, if she stopped drinking coffee and eating muffins altogether, but until she's ready to make that change, she substitutes a healthier alternative. At least she has made one small step. The pyramids were built of individual blocks of stone. Mrs. L. has added one more block to the structure of her new life.

Exhibit 3–5
Finding Substitutes

High-Risk Foods	Substitutions
cheese cake, chocolate cake, apple pastries, doughnuts	angel food cake, muffins, pie without crust, fresh fruit, bagels, cinnamon raisinbread, low-fat cookies (e.g.,Fig Newtons, gingersnaps, or graham crackers)
potato chips, nacho chips, cheese twists, peanuts	melba toast, low-fat biscuits with salsa, rice crackers, popcorn (no butter, light salt), pretzels, roasted chestnuts
ice cream sundaes or milkshakes	low-fat frozen yogurt, sherbets, frozen fruit ices, drinks such as Appeal®, Enercal®, Ensure Plus®
chocolate bars	licorice, jujubes, raisins, gumdrops, jelly beans, more nutritional bars such asBreakbar®,Fiberry®, PowerBar®, Exceed®
hamburgers, hot dogs, fried fast foods butter, mayonnaise, margarine	barbecued chicken sandwich with salad, rice, or baked potatoes whole-fruit jam, flavored mustard, low-fat cheese

If you are able to completely eliminate unhealthy foods, that's great. If not, look for a less harmful substitution.

Do you have a job that requires you to travel or a job that often leaves you with little time for lunch? If you don't plan a proper lunch for yourself, you may find that when hunger hits you, you look for the nearest fast-food restaurant. In this moment of weakness and low blood sugar, you can easily revert to the burger-and-fries mentality.

If you find yourself in this situation, you can make health-promoting substitutions. Many restaurants have expanded their menus to meet the needs of the growing wellness-oriented market. A barbecued or grilled (not fried) chicken sandwich with lettuce and tomatoes and a baked potato is an excellent substitution for a hamburger with French fries or onion rings. Food is part of what makes life interesting and enjoyable, but it is in your best interest to find foods that are satisfying without being disease-promoting. In almost any situation, you can step back from temptation and make a less damaging food choice.

From our experience, we know that you are more likely to succeed with the Winning Weigh if you try to find agreeable substitutions rather than just eliminating your favorite foods. If you're suddenly faced with a dessert tray of gooey, killer foods such as cherry cheesecake or "death by chocolate" pastries, you will probably find it rather difficult to skip dessert entirely. Instead of depriving yourself, select a less damaging dessert like sherbet or a frozen fruit ice. If you make this choice consistently, you can allow yourself the odd gooey treat without feeling guilty.

We've convinced many of our friends to eat high-fiber biscuits and salsa sauce instead of potato chips and sour cream dip. Unbuttered popcorn, pita and bagel chips, fresh fruit, and low-fat yogurt with whole-fruit jam are also excellent choices.

Nutritional supplements are an increasingly popular way to acquire a concentrated dose of many essential nutrients. These supplements are available as drinks or bars. The drinks have the consistency of milkshakes but contain much less fat. They generally satisfy your appetite. If you are an athlete, they provide an easy way to conveniently increase carbohydrate loading and also enhance your lean body mass with a generous protein contribution. You can use these products as meal replacements when you are trying to control your weight. Meal substitutes are also handy for busy executives who want a healthy alternative to fast foods.

Exhibits 3-6 and 3-8 show some of the nutritional content of some popular nutritional supplements.

Exhibit 3-6
Nutritional Supplement Drinks

	Appeal® Nu Skin International Inc.	Enercal® Wyeth Ltd.	Ensure Plus® Ross Laboratories, Division of Abbott Lab Ltd.
Serving size	56 g (230 ml)	240 ml	235 ml
Calories	227 cal.	240 cal.	355 cal.
Protein	15 g	9.5 g	12.9 g
Carbohydrates	35 g	32.6 g	47 g
Fat	3 g	8.1 g	12.5 g
Sodium	250 mg	120 mg	248 mg
Potassium	390 mg	300 mg	446 mg
Vitamin A	450 I.U.	800 I.U.	505.3 I.U.
Vitamin D	2 µg	64 I.U.	35.25 I.U.
Vitamin E	4 mg	4.8 I.U.	7.8 I.U.
Vitamin C	15 mg	32 mg	49.7 mg
Vitamin B_1	375 µg	0.21 mg	0.5 mg
Vitamin B_2	375 µg	0.29 mg	0.57 mg
Niacin	5.5 mg	3.2 mg	6.63 mg
Vitamin B_6	0.675 mg	0.31 mg	0.67 mg
Vitamin B_{12}	0.4 µg	0.96 µg	0.002 mg
Pantothenic acid	2 mg	1.6 mg	3.32 mg
Biotin	0.025 µg	48 µg	0.09 mg
Folic acid	100 µg	64 µg	0.13 mg
Calcium	360 mg	154 mg	149 mg
Magnesium	75 mg	64 mg	74.5 mg
Iron	4 mg	2.9 mg	2.98 mg
Zinc	5 mg	2.4 mg	3.72 mg

The Emergency Snack

What if you are hungry at a time when there are no Winning Weigh foods around? Even the most dedicated may surrender in the face of escalating hunger. How do you deal with business meetings or seminars where doughnuts and pastries are provided as the mid-morning or afternoon snack? What if you're driving all over town with a hundred errands to do and you only have time for a quick bite to eat?

The solution is to prepare for those moments of weakness. Carry an emergency snack with you in case hunger strikes in a situation where a Winning Weigh meal is impractical. Keep it in your backpack, purse, briefcase, or desk drawer. Any easily-transportable complex carbohydrate food will do. By snacking in this manner, you can restore normal blood sugar levels at vulnerable moments during the day, staving off hunger until you can find the time to sit down to a proper Winning Weigh meal.

Exhibit 3–7
Complex Carbohydrate Snacks

- fresh fruit
- dried fruit
- crackers
- raw vegetable sticks
- unbuttered popcorn
- muffins (occasionally)

In addition to foods such as raw fruits and vegetables, new nutritional snacks are appearing on the market. These bars have a lower fat content than traditional snack foods. They are also enriched with health-promoting nutrients such as fiber, calcium, and iron. As you can see in Exhibit 3–8, this new generation of snacks offers healthy alternatives to traditional chocolate bars.It only takes a few minutes a day to prepare an emergency snack. You'll be glad you did. Planning ahead of time is a major way of staying on the wellness track.

Exhibit 3–8
Snack Bars
(not all nutrients have been listed in this table)

	Typical Chocolate Bar	French Muesli Breakbar® Interior Design Nutritionals	Power Bar ® Meal Replacement	Nature's Plus® Spiru-tein High Protein Energy Meal	Nectar Granola Bar® Natural Nectar Corporation
Amount[1]	1 bar (66.5 g)	1 bar (57 g)	1 bar (65 g)	1 bar (39 g)	1 bar (34 g)
Calories	330 cal.	180 cal.	225 cal.	159 cal.	120 cal.
Protein	7.5 g	7 g	12 g	10 g	2 g
Carbohydrates	38 g	38 g	37.5 g	21 g	20 g
Fat	17 g	4 g*	3 g*	4 g*	4 g*
Fiber	Not listed	6 g*	Not listed	3 g*	6 g*
Sodium	45 g	80 mg	250 mg	80 mg	30 mg
Potassium	210 g	130 mg	375 mg	45 mg	100 mg
Calcium	Not listed	100 mg*	288 mg*	240 mg*	Not listed
Magnesium	Not listed	7.5 mg	210 mg	52.5 mg	Not listed
Zinc	Not listed	2.25 mg*	8.25 mg*	2.25 mg*	Not listed
Iron	Not listed	3.6 mg*	5 mg*	5 mg*	Not listed

[1] Note that bars vary in size.
* Significant attributes compared to typical chocolate bars.

A Typical Day with the Winning Weigh

Our patients and clients often ask us what *we*, as doctors and firm believers in the Winning Weigh program, eat for breakfast or make for dinner. They want to know how we make the program work for *us*. So we thought we'd give you an idea of how we manage to stay on track.

Breakfast is a low-fat, high-fiber meal. We start with six to ten ounces of low-fat yogurt, to which we add about 1/2 cup of bran cereal and 2 tablespoons of oat bran. We might add some slices of honeydew melon, peaches, or other fruit to give it some flavor and wash it down with a glass of fruit juice, diluted with pure spring water. The yogurt is an excellent source of protein, calcium, and vitamin D. The bran cereal contains colon cleaner fiber and enough complex carbohydrates to kick-start our day. The oat bran helps keep our cholesterol levels low.

For lunch we might choose a low-fat flesh-protein meal such as steamed rice with stir-fried vegetables and pieces of chicken or shrimp. We try to choose vegetables that are rich in anti-cancer nutrients, such as broccoli or carrots.

For our complex-carbohydrate-only dinner, we often eat a plate of fresh pasta with lightly seasoned tomato sauce, a salad with olive oil and vinegar dressing, and a whole wheat roll.

We usually have fresh fruit for a snack, but low-fat, high-fiber cookies sometimes appear in our food diaries, which we still keep faithfully.

Starting Right Now . . .

1. Prepare an emergency snack for all those places you might get caught without wellness alternatives to high-fat, disease-promoting foods – your home, your office, your car, your briefcase, your purse.

2. Eat no more than one Compromise Food per day and no more than one or two Recreational Foods per week.

3. Cross Hazardous Foods off your shopping list.

4. In the Wellness Planner, list all the Recreational and Hazardous Foods you eat now. Find some Winning Weigh substitutions from the Wellness or Compromise Foods to eat instead.

Food Preparation Guide
General Tips

When shopping, try to choose foods with three or fewer grams of fat per 100 calories. Each gram of fat has 9 calories, so the calories you get from fat from these foods would be almost ideal – about 27 percent of the total.

- Non-stick pans enable you to cook without adding extra fat. If you have ordinary pans, use a non-stick spray instead of greasing them.
- Low-fat cooking doesn't have to be tasteless. Experiment with herbs and spices. Add them to soups, casseroles, pasta, salads, and popcorn.
- Prepare food in ways that don't require added oil. Try broiling, baking, microwaving, or steaming.
- Sauté in wine or broth instead of oil.

Low-Fat Flesh Protein Foods

- Broil, grill, or steam poultry and fish.
- Cook poultry and fish in a fondue, using consommé broth or a clear broth instead of oil.
- Poach poultry and fish in clear broth, vegetable juices, or water seasoned with lemon.
- Barbecue chicken or, occasionally, low-fat ground beef.
- Take the skin off chicken, preferably before cooking it. Choose white rather than dark meat.

- When roasting chicken or turkey, baste with broth instead of fatty drippings.

- If you do occasionally eat red meat, buy lean cuts and trim off all excess fat.

- The fish highest in Omega 3 fats are salmon, mackerel, herring, trout, sardines, shad, anchovies, and albacore tuna. Clams, crab, and mussels also contain Omega 3 fats.

- Add seafood, such as clams or mussels, to pasta dishes. Linguine alla vongole ("with clam sauce") is delicious.

- Choose water-packed, not oil-packed, canned fish. Rinse the salt off canned fish.

- Mix tuna or salmon salad with yogurt instead of mayonnaise.

- Frozen dinners that are labelled "light" or "low-calorie" are not necessarily low in fat. Read the label carefully and choose only those that have fewer than 10 grams of fat per 300-calorie serving.

Low-Fat Dairy Protein

- Drink milk with no more than 1% M.F.

- Eat plain yogurt that contains 1% M.F. or less. Avoid flavored and presweetened yogurt. You can make your own flavors by adding fresh fruit, whole-fruit jam, wheat germ, Winning Weigh Fiber Mixture, or cereal.

- Eat cheese with 10% M.F. or less. Also, try to find cheese that is low in salt. Most solid cheeses are more than 25% M.F. Cheddar, for example, is 32% M.F., and brick is 29% M.F.

- Try some low-fat cheeses such as ricotta, low-fat cottage cheese, low-fat mozzarella, farmer's cheese, any skim milk cheese, or low-fat cream cheese.

- If you order pizza, order only half the regular amount of cheese. Avoid high-fat toppings such as bacon, sausage, pepperoni, and olives. Even better – buy a pizza shell or plain frozen pizza and add your own vegetable toppings.

- Try buttermilk made from skim milk.

- Spread low-fat cheese thinly on bread as a substitute for butter or margarine.

- If you really dislike black coffee, use low-fat milk instead of cream or non-dairy creamer. Refer to the Fiber Scoreboard (pp. 294-303) for other selections.

Breakfast Cereals

- Choose cereals that are unsweetened and high in fiber. Some good brands and types are Kelloggs All-Bran, Post Grape Nuts, Bran Flakes, Bran Buds, Nabisco 100% Bran, Shredded Wheat, Special K, Wheeta Bix, Quaker Puffed Wheat or Puffed Rice, oatmeal, and muesli. Refer to the Fiber Scoreboard (pp. 294-303) for other selections.

Bread

- Choose bread that is high in natural fiber but low in fat: whole wheat, pumpernickel, rye, whole wheat bagels, and pita.

- Toasting bread increases its fiber content.

- Don't butter your bread. Butter is 80 percent fat. You should also try to avoid margarine.

- Whole fruit jam is a good alternative to butter. Read the label to be sure it is high in fruit and low in sugar. Jam spread thinly on bread counts as one serving of complex carbohydrates.

- Spread low-fat cheese on your bread for a low-fat dairy meal.

- Avoid egg breads and bread products that are high in saturated fats.

- Try making yogurt "cheese" by taking low-fat yogurt and letting it drain through a fine sieve or a piece of cheesecloth overnight.

Crackers and Biscuits

- Many crackers are made with palm or coconut oil. Avoid these types. Some healthy choices are rice crackers, bread sticks, melba toast, soda crackers, and matzoth.

- Avoid all fried biscuits, chips, nachos, and tortillas, regardless of the kind of oil they were fried in. Not only are they high in total fat, but the oil they were fried in may have been heated to high temperatures and left exposed to light and air, causing it to become carcinogenic.

- For snacks, try baked, crispy bread products, such as pita chips and bagel chips.

- Fiber cookies, often available at drug stores, also make a great, crunchy snack.

Fruit

- All kinds of fruit are good for you.

- The best cholesterol-lowering fruits are apples, peaches, pears, plums, nectarines, the white rind of citrus fruits, blueberries, strawberries, raspberries, mangoes, and papaya.

- Anti-cancer fruits are those with lots of vitamin C or beta-carotene. Citrus fruits and kiwis have the most vitamin C. Orange fruits, including cantaloupe, apricots, peaches, nectarines, oranges, mangoes, and watermelon, are highest in beta-carotene.

- Fruit salad makes a wonderful dessert.

Vegetables

- You should eat a wide variety of vegetables, choosing them as your complex carbohydrates as often as possible.

- Cruciferous vegetables include Brussels sprouts, cabbage, turnips, cauliflower, and broccoli. They are good anti-cancer foods.

- Vegetables high in beta-carotene are also good anti-cancer foods. Carrots, squash, eggplant, and other orange/yellow vegetables, broccoli, spinach, and dark green, leafy vegetables are all high in beta-carotene.

- Try vegetables raw, steamed, broiled, microwaved, marinated, or stir-fried. Serve them with rice.

- Carrots, potatoes, and peas are high in cholesterol cruncher fiber, so they are especially good for your heart.

- Bake or boil potatoes. Do not add butter; use low-fat yogurt (1% M.F.) or ultra low-fat sour cream (3% to

5% M.F.). Try eating baked potatoes without adding anything. Give your taste buds a chance to explore.

- Avocadoes are high in monounsaturated fat (the same kind of fat found in olive and peanut oils). However, they are also high in vitamins and minerals, so you may eat small amounts occasionally. Try two small slices in a sandwich along with tomatoes, cucumbers, and alfalfa sprouts. A little bit of avocado is a good substitute for cheese and other animal-based foods.

- Salads are a heathy way to eat vegetables. Spinach salad, chef's salad, and mixed green salads, tossed with a light olive oil and vinegar dressing, are the best options. Shredded cabbage, seasoned with a light olive oil and vinegar dressing, is a tasty alternative to lettuce. Caesar salad is all right for a change, but don't add bacon or Parmesan cheese. Greek salads are definitely bad: feta cheese is loaded with both fat and salt and hard-boiled eggs are high in cholesterol.

- Try flavored vinegars to add variety to your salads. You can purchase them or make your own by dropping fresh herbs or garlic into wine vinegar and letting the mixture sit for a week.

Grains

- Rice is best steamed or boiled.

- Brown rice is better than white rice because of its high fiber content.

Peas and Beans

- If you are using canned peas or beans, put them in a strainer and rinse with water to get rid of the excess salt and oil.

- If you are cooking dried beans yourself, completely cover them with cold water overnight. The next day, drain them and cook in fresh water until they are tender.

- Peas and beans are perfectly balanced foods. Most are 60 percent complex carbohydrates, 15 percent protein, and 25 percent fat – precisely in tune with your genetic dietary requirements and the overall formula of the Winning Weigh program.

Pasta

- All noodles are acceptable, but egg noodles are higher in cholesterol.

- Whole wheat noodles and spinach noodles are especially good choices.

- Gnocchi, made from potatoes and flour, are another good option. They are a good source of protein, low in fat, and high in complex carbohydrates.

- Use light (low-fat) tomato sauces. Sauté vegetables in water or olive oil to add to the sauce. Green peppers, red peppers, mushrooms, onions, and zucchini are all excellent choices. Add clams, mussels, scallops, or chicken to your tomato sauce too, if you wish.

- Do not use cream sauces or meat sauces. They are very high in fat.

- Bottled tomato sauces with meat are also high in fat. Go to the refrigerator section of the grocery store and buy a fresh marinara sauce and add your own fresh vegetables. The vegetables will improve the taste, add vitamins, and dilute the fat content.

Oils

- Use olive oil for salad dressings or for sautéing vegetables.

- Use peanut oil for stir frying.

- Vegetable oil sprays (such as Pam®) are acceptable substitutes for vegetable oils.

- Use fat-free, butter-flavored sprinkles instead of butter, margarine, or oil.

Snack Foods and Desserts

- The urge to eat dessert is often a result of delayed satiety after the meal you have just eaten. It takes more than 30 minutes for your brain's appetite center to shut off. So wait for 10 to 15 minutes after a meal before deciding to indulge in a dessert. You will probably find that you are satisfied and no longer crave a treat.

- Get up from the table before dessert is served and go for a walk. This will curb your appetite and help you digest your meal.

- Unbuttered popcorn is a good snack food. Popcorn made in an air popper has the least amount of fat. Most microwave popcorn is high in fat. Try using a salt substitute, too.

- Munchies such as potato chips, nacho chips, and cheezies are very high in fat.

- For healthy munchies try melba toast with salsa, rice crackers, raisins, baked bagel slices, or low-fat biscuits.

- Bran, oatmeal, or blueberry muffins are better options than doughnuts.

- If you are a dessert lover, plan to have dessert once a week so you don't feel deprived or unrewarded for your day-to-day efforts. Choose your moments carefully and don't overdo it. Sherbets, fruit ices, and frozen tofu desserts are all good options. You can also eat low-fat frozen yogurt or even ice cream once in awhile. The best dessert for you, of course, is fresh fruit.

- Make your own chips. Cut corn tortillas into pieces, lightly coat a baking dish with non-stick spray, and bake at 375° F (200°C) until they are light brown and crunchy.

Beverages

- Every day, you should drink six to eight glasses of water. Distilled water, spring water, low-sodium mineral water and soda water are all good choices.

- Bottled water should be ozone-treated to help prevent bacterial growth. The best water is either distilled or has undergone reverse osmosis and deionization.

- As a complex carbohydrate selection, you can dilute 1/4 glass of unsweetened juice with 3/4 glass of water or soda water.

- Keep your intake of caffeinated beverages to a minimum. Two cups of coffee a day should be your maximum. Drink it black.

- Try herbal teas or hot water and lemon as an alternative to coffee or regular tea.

- Diet drinks that contain aspartame are the most acceptable soft drinks, but don't overdo it. There is no nutritional value whatsoever in diet soft drinks.

- Avoid all beverages sweetened with sugar.

- Beware of high-sodium drinks. They make your body retain sodium and water, creating a bloating effect. They also impair your body's ability to rid itself of toxins and metabolic debris.

- Tap water is always an unknown quantity. It might be wise to attach a water purifier to your water tap. Reduce the amount of tap water you drink by as much as possible.

- The occasional alcoholic beverage is acceptable, but moderation is the key.

- You can increase the amount of fluids you get by eating foods that have a high water content. The following foods contain more than 80 percent water: lettuce, celery, broccoli, collards, snap beans, watermelon, carrots, skim milk, radishes, raw cabbage, beets, oranges, grapefruit, and tangerines.

Dining at Restaurants

- Ask for your meal to be prepared with less fat than the chef would normally use. In Chinese restaurants, for example, ask the waiter to reduce the amount of oil used for stir frying.

- When travelling by plane, call ahead to request a low-fat meal or go for the vegetarian option.

- Salad bars are filled with high-fat extras, such as bacon bits, egg yolks, olives, and potato salads. Avoid these foods, concentrating on the fresh vegetables.

- Ask for creamy sauces and dressings to be served on the side. This way you can control how much you will use, if any.

- Order baked potatoes, rice, or pasta instead of fries.

- At Mexican fast-food outlets, order plain bean tostadas or bean burritos. At hamburger places, order fish or chicken sandwiches without the sauce. (Be sure that they are grilled, not fried.)

Here are a few examples of good food selections from a number of different types of restaurants:

Chinese Restaurants

Our favorite is Moo Goo Gai Pan – a bed of steamed rice covered with stir-fried vegetables (broccoli, onions, Swiss chard, Chinese vegetables, carrots, etc.) and shrimp or chicken. You might also want to try:

    vegetable chow mein or chop suey
    orange chicken
    shrimps in garlic or tomato sauce

Avoid fried dishes, especially foods in batter such as chicken balls or lemon chicken. Pork selections are off limits.

Italian Restaurants

As an appetizer, try
    minestrone soup
    radicchio salad, with the dressing on the side
    mixed green salad (insalata mista), dressing on the side
    tomato and bocconcino cheese
    calamari salad, oil dressing on the side

For the main course, consider
    pasta in red sauce (e.g., spaghetti pomadoro)
    pasta with seafood in a red sauce (e.g., linguine pescatore or vongole)
    penne arrabbiata

any grilled fish or chicken

pizza, with half the normal amount of cheese. Ask what percentage of milk fat is listed for the cheese they are using; be sure it is 10% M.F. or less. Add vegetarian toppings of your choice.

Mexican Restaurants

Our favorites are chicken faijites, made with stir-fried chicken and onion. You can then make into a Mexican sandwich by rolling chicken, onions, and other vegetables with salsa sauce in a soft tortilla bread. Leave out the sour cream and guacamole – they would add too much fat. Bean burritos, if you leave out the cheese, are also quite low in fat.

Chicken Restaurants

chicken breast (grilled or barbecued), with skin removed
baked potato or rice, no French fries (have the potato without butter or margarine)
whole wheat roll (no butter)

Deli or Greasy Spoon Dining

turkey sandwich on whole wheat, pumpernickel, or rye bread (add tomato, lettuce, and even mustard for moisture, but no butter, margarine, or mayonnaise)
chicken breast sandwich (same rules as above)
single serving of canned salmon or tuna on a plate (no mayonnaise)
toasted bagel or bread (no butter or margarine)
mixed salad, dressing on the side
vegetable, pea, or minestrone soup
pancakes, instead of waffles or bacon and eggs (use just a little syrup, but no butter; buckwheat pancakes are the healthiest)

Fast-Food Restaurants
   salad bar
   grilled or barbecued chicken

Combination Foods

We have tried to keep the Winning Weigh program simple. Some confusion may result, however, when you have prepared dishes with more than one main ingredient. We call these combination foods. Pizza, lasagna, cabbage rolls, and stuffed peppers, for example, all contain both protein and complex carbohydrates. You need to count them as both protein and complex carbohydrates when you record them in your journal.

You will get into trouble, however, when a dish contains both dairy and flesh foods. Traditional lasagna is a good example of a double trouble food – it contains both high-fat beef and high-fat cheese. As a general rule, try not to eat a dairy protein at the same meal as a flesh protein. Divide your daily consumption of protein between two meals. That way, your body will be able to better assimilate the protein as it needs it. If you ingest too much protein at one time, you risk overloading your body's capacity to use protein efficiently. As a result, some of the excess protein may be converted into fats and carbohydrates, leaving damaging by-products in your system. Here are some examples of healthy foods that combine protein and complex carbohydrates. Because they all contain one low-fat dairy or flesh protein and at least two different complex carbohydrates, they satisfy the formula for a protein meal all by themselves:

- Italian manicotta: tubular pasta noodles stuffed with low-fat ricotta cheese and cooked spinach, covered with seasoned tomato sauce and baked.

- vegetarian pizza: pizza dough, covered with low-fat mozzarella cheese and tomato sauce. Additional toppings can include green peppers, mushrooms, onions, sliced tomatoes, and red peppers.

- vegetarian lasagna: pasta noodles baked with low-fat ricotta or mozzarella cheese, tomato sauce, and additional vegetables, such as spinach and mushrooms.

- stuffed tomatoes: baked tomatoes stuffed with low-fat cheese and spinach.

- cabbage rolls: boiled cabbage stuffed with rice, tomatoes, and optional lean ground veal or turkey.

- stuffed green peppers: baked green peppers stuffed with rice, tomatoes, and optional lean ground veal or turkey.

- stir fry: small chunks of chicken breast or seafood and assorted vegetables (e.g., broccoli, peppers, onions, green beans, zucchini, and cabbage) stir fried in peanut oil and served over a bed of steamed rice.

- seafood and pasta salad: cooked pasta (usually rotini or shells), served cold with crab meat or shrimp, lightly seasoned with an olive oil or vinegar dressing.

- soup: vegetable, minestrone, cabbage borscht, matzoh balls, chicken noodle and other broth- or tomato-based soups are fantastic complex carbohydrate foods. They help fill up your stomach and are a pleasant change from salads. Be careful of commercially-prepared soups, however. They usually have a very high sodium content. Cream-based soups are definitely not a good idea, since they are very high in fat.

- pasta fagioli: pasta and beans

- ratatouille served with rice

- tuna and vegetable salad: chunks of water-packed tuna served on a bed of mixed salad vegetables and dressed with olive oil and vinegar

Recipes

You probably know the saying, "Give a man a fish and feed him for a day, or teach him how to fish and feed him for a lifetime." The Winning Weigh is about learning how to fish, and how to feed yourself in a health-promoting way for a lifetime. Now that you know the rules of the game, you should be able to look at any recipe and know whether or not it meets the requirements of the Winning Weigh program. If the recipe doesn't meet your needs, you may be able to adapt it.

We have encountered a number of excellent cookbooks that are loaded with recipes that fit the Winning Weigh lifestyle. We have included a few favorites for you in the next section. You may be surprised at how many of your own favorite recipes you can adapt to fit the Winning Weigh program. Here are some tips:

- Cut back (by as much as half) on the amount of fat called for in a recipe. Usually, you won't miss it at all. This is especially true for the amount of oil needed to sauté vegetables.

- Try thickening sauces and soups with mashed potatoes, puréed beans, or cornstarch dissolved in water.

- Instead of sautéing onions before adding them to food, chop them and cook them in the microwave oven for about 30 seconds.

- Replace all butter with olive oil or peanut oil.

- Substitute yogurt for sour cream or mayonnaise.

- Substitute skinned chicken for beef or pork.

- For muffins or quick breads, substitute applesauce for the same amount of oil or butter. They will still be moist and delicious.

- Substitute two egg whites for each whole egg in a recipe.

- Use evaporated skim milk instead of cream in sauces and desserts.

Your First Winning Weigh Shopping List

If you are serious about eating more healthy foods, you can start by doing two simple things. First, prepare a shopping list of foods that are included on the Winning Weigh program and stockpile them in your home. That way you will always have Winning Weigh foods close at hand.

Second, stop buying foods that will tempt you into failure, such as potato chips, cakes, pies, pastries, ice cream, candy, cookies, and chocolate. Remember the principle of "out of sight, out of mind." Don't rationalize by telling yourself that you are buying these items for company, for the kids, or for your spouse. If you really care about them, you'll encourage them to follow the Winning Weigh program too. If you don't buy junk food in the first place, you won't be tempted by it.

To help you get started, we have prepared a shopping list that you can use to fill your home with Winning Weigh foods. Under each category, choose the foods that you like the best.

Beverages

- A variety of pure fruit and/or vegetable juices, with no added sugar (juice concentrates are okay as long as they are not sweetened)

- Pure spring water, distilled water

- Low-sodium mineral water and/or low-sodium soda water

- Diet drinks

- Other no-calorie beverages, such as herbal tea

Fruits and Vegetables

- A variety of fresh fruit (Try to choose ones that are high in vitamin C, beta-carotene, and/or cholesterol cruncher fiber. Fruits such as grapes and cherries have fewer benefits.)

- Lemons (Squeeze lemon into a cup of water; serve hot or cold.)

- Canned or frozen fruit packed in its own juice, without added sugar

- Dried fruits, including raisins, for between-meal snacks

- A variety of fresh vegetables (Focus on vegetables that are high in fiber and anti-cancer nutrients.)

- Salad vegetables

- Vegetables, such as carrots, that can be cut into sticks for snacks

- Potatoes

- Canned tomatoes (for pasta)

- Frozen vegetables, without added sodium

Bread Products

- Whole grain breads and rolls, including wheat, rye, and pumpernickel (Focus on products that are high in fiber and low in fat.)

- High-fiber, low-fat biscuits

- Bagels

- Melba toast, rice crackers, bread sticks, soda crackers, and matzoth

- Pizza dough

- Low-fat muffins
- Pita bread
- Fiber cookies
- Baked pita and bagel chips

Cereals and Grains
- High-fiber breakfast cereals
- Oat bran and wheat bran
- Wheat germ
- Rice and other grains
- Pasta and noodles, preferably spinach or whole wheat

Legumes
- A variety of peas and beans, especially chick-peas and red kidney beans

Low-Fat Flesh Proteins
- chicken breasts
- cooked, sliced chicken or turkey breast for sandwiches
- Turkey (white meat)
- Cornish game hens
- Fresh or frozen fish, preferably varieties high in Omega 3 fats such as mackerel, halibut, sardines, and salmon
- Canned water-packed salmon and tuna
- Other kinds of seafood, such as clams, crab, mussels, and shrimp

Low-Fat Dairy Protein
- Plain yogurt with no more than 1% M.F.
- Skim milk or milk with 1% M.F.
- Low-fat cheese (under 10% M.F.)

Miscellaneous
- Popcorn
- Tomato sauce (for pasta)
- Extra virgin olive oil
- Peanut oil
- Vegetable oil sprays
- A variety of herbs and spices
- Vinegar
- Whole-fruit or dietetic jam, low in added sugar
- Salsa sauce
- Low-sodium clear broth and legume soups
- Vegetarian alternatives, such as miso, tofu, soy milk, and tempeh

Occasional Foods
- Avocadoes
- Diet soda drinks
- Frozen fruit ices or sherbets
- Low-fat frozen yogurt
- Pretzels (low sodium)
- Lean beef or veal
- Margarine

Starting Right Now . . .

1. Prepare a Winning Weigh shopping list. Then go out and stock your home full of wellness foods. Remember: out of sight, out of mind!
2. Go through all your recipes to see which ones you can adapt to your new wellness lifestyle. Throw out the ones that you can't adapt – if you don't have them, you won't use them!
3. Purchase or borrow some wellness-oriented cookbooks. Go through them and find some recipes you want to try. Start a file of Winning Weigh recipes clipped from magazines and newspapers.
4. In your Wellness Planner, write down the preparation hints that you will now incorporate into your cooking style.

Future Trends: Designer Foods and Supplements

Numerous studies published in the past few years have concluded that individuals with higher lifetime intakes and blood levels of beta-carotene, vitamin C, and vitamin E develop significantly fewer cancers than individuals with less intake and lower blood levels. Unfortunately, because of poor eating habits, only 9 percent of our population attain the recommended dietary allowances for all nutrients.

In her book, ***The Popcorn Report***, future trend forecaster Faith Popcorn predicts that as people realize that good health extends life, there will be new products, a new emphasis on fitness, and a new way of life.

She suggests that "foodaceuticals," or designer foods, will blend health-promoting nutrients, such as anti-oxidants, into specialized foods that will enhance life. A number of food companies are beginning to produce a new generation of designer food lines and products. These products are a healthy alternative to what people typically consume. Generally, these food products are low in fat (including saturated fat and cholesterol), provide generous quantities of fiber, and are enriched with anti-oxidant nutrients like beta-carotene, vitamin C, and vitamin E. Various minerals, such as calcium, iron, zinc, and selenium may be included in safe doses to help balance out common dietary deficiencies.

We live in a fast-paced world in which we are growing increasingly dependent on fast foods and convenience foods. This pattern will not change. What has changed, however, is that new designer foods, which are fast and convenient, are becoming healthy alternatives to burgers, milk shakes, chocolate bars, doughnuts, and soft drinks. Many companies are now producing alternative foods that are designed to enhance health not detract from it. It is now easier to adopt a diet low in fat, high in complex carbohydrates, high in fiber, and enriched with many protective nutrients and essential minerals.

A growing body of research demonstrates that vitamin and mineral supplementation in strategic doses will help to prevent or retard disease. Presently, the National Cancer Institute is conducting 21 studies using nutrients like beta-carotene. Many health authorities are currently suggesting that supplementation would correct some of the poor dietary habits that we see and could be a safe and practical way to help people get their blood levels of beta-carotene, vitamin C, and vitamin E into safer ranges.

The Argument in Favor of Vitamin and Mineral Supplementation

In 1979, Hirayama published the first prospective study that revealed an association between vegetable and fruit consumption and reduction in cancer risk. Since this first report, an additional five major prospective studies have examined the same relationship. Researchers have indentified a number of nutrients in various vegetables and fruits that appear to offer a considerable degree of protection against a number of cancers. Orange-yellow vegetables and fruits contain beta-carotene and other related compounds known as *carotenoids.* Beta-carotene and a few other carotenoids we now recognize exert a number of anti-cancer effects. Most of the ongoing research, however, has been aimed at beta-carotene specifically.

People with higher blood levels of beta-carotene have a significantly lower chance of developing certain cancers. Beta-carotene appears to exert its anti-cancer effects by quenching free radicals, strengthening the immune system, and even reversing some precancerous states. People can raise their blood levels of beta-carotene by simply ingesting more foods that contain the nutrient or by taking beta-carotene in supplement form.

Unfortunately, the average dietary intake of beta-carotene in our society is four times lower than that recommended by governmental authorities. The average intake level of beta-carotene from food stands at approximately 2500 I.U. per day. Government health authorities in the United States recommend an intake of approximately 10,000 I.U. per day. In his book, **Cancer and Nutrition,** Dr. Charles B. Simone recommends an intake of beta-carotene at a level of 25,000 I.U. per day as a cancer-prevention strategy.

As we mentioned earlier, vitamin C and vitamin E also quench free radicals and are thereby associated with decreased cancer risk. However, studies suggest that intake levels needed to protect against cancer exceed what we are used to seeing as recommended daily allowances. For instance, the recommended daily allowance for vitamin C is 60 mg, a dose that will defend against the development of scurvy. An intake level this low doesn't seem to provide as much protection from the risk of cancer as higher levels would.

In view of studies that have been done and with the evidence that the vitamin C turnover rate in the body is increasing today as our bodies try to block nitrosamine formation, quench toxic air pollutant agents such as ozone and nitrogen oxide, and, possibly, reduce the binding of cancer-causing agents to genetic material, it seems necessary to consume vitamin C in larger daily quantities than 60 mg. As well, cigarette smoking substantially increases the turnover of vitamin C. Smokers are particularly known for their lower blood levels of vitamin C and beta-carotene and therefore have a higher requirement for both nutrients.

Studies that provide individuals with supplements of vitamin C have been shown to decrease cancer-causing chemicals in fecal matter, to minimize lung damage in the presence of various contaminants and free radicals, and to boost immune system function. In light of all of these findings, many health authorities are recommending daily vitamin C supplementation in the range of 250 mg to 2,000 mg, depending on individual lifestyle factors as well as family and medical history. (People who have had kidney stones or any history of kidney disease should not take vitamin C supplements.)

In the case of vitamin E, the usual recommended daily allowance stands at 15 I.U. This level is far below what is required in order to derive any significant protection against cancer of the lungs, stomach, pancreas, colon, and reproductive organs.

Various studies demonstrate that vitamin E supplementation greatly minimizes free radicle damage to lung tissue. Evidence also shows that vitamin E supplementation enhances immune system function, even in elderly subjects. Vitamin E also blocks the formation of cancer-causing nitrosamines in the stomach.

Another attractive feature of vitamin E supplementation is that it has been shown to decrease the stickiness of blood platelets. Additionally, vitamin E in the bloodstream protects cholesterol from free radicle damage. Cholesterol that is damaged by free radicles is much more inclined to stick to the walls of your arteries and cause accelerated narrowing, which can lead to a stroke or heart attack.

While we may benefit from a daily intake higher than 15 I.U., it is extremely difficult to attain more optimal levels of vitamin E from food sources alone. Daily supplementation of vitamin E is likely to be the most practical and effective option. Many health authorities recommend a dose of 100 I.U. to 400 I.U. of vitamin E per day, taken with food to ensure absorption. (People taking anti-coagulant medication should not take vitamin E supplementation.)

From the total body evidence available today, it seems reasonable to consider taking additional amounts of anti-oxidants, beta-carotene, vitamin C, and vitamin E, over and above the nutrition provided by Winning Weigh foods. These vitamins are extremely non-toxic, and their potential benefits in the area of cancer prevention, enhanced immune system function, lowered risk of cardiovascular disease, and increased longevity make them very desirable as supplemental nutrients. As it is still quite debatable what vitamin doses represent an ideal intake, a cautious approach for most people might include

Vitamin C	250-500 mg
Beta-carotene	10,000 mg (25,000 I.U.)
Vitamin E	100-400 I.U.

Vitamin A is also known to be a powerful anti-cancer nutrient, but it is also potentially toxic at doses as low as 10,000 to

20,000 I.U. Therefore, if you take a multiple vitamin and mineral supplement, it is our opinion that it should contain no more than 7500 I.U. of vitamin A.

Recently, two new anti-oxidant nutrients have been introduced to the marketplace. Glutathione and Pycnogenol are both very powerful quenchers of free radicles and are now included in several superior multiple vitamin and mineral supplements.

Most people today would not dream of lying out in the sun without applying suntan lotion to block damaging ultra-violet radiation. Ultraviolet light damages the skin and the melanocytes below the skin through free radicle attack; suntan lotions contain agents that help block free radicle attack of the skin. By the same token, the inside of the body requires adequate amounts of anti-oxidants in order to quench the increasing number of free radicle agents to which our tissues are continually being exposed. The following list contains some of the environmental agents that generate free radicles in the body:

Benzopyrene, from automobile emissions, industrial waste, smoked foods and barbequed meats
Nitrosamines, from meats preserved with nitrate salts and from the increased levels of nitrates in vegetables and water supplies due to the use of nitrogen fertilizers
Chlorinated particles, formed in water supplies as a feature of the chlorination process to control microorganisms
Ground-level ozone, generated from automobile emissions and industrial waste
Nitrogen oxide, an additional component of photochemical smog that damages lung tissue

All of these chemicals, which have become more apparent in recent years, are known to cause free-radical damage to the body and are thus potential carcinogens. Some other occupational and environmental carcinogens are listed in Exhibit 3–9.

Exhibit 3-9
Carcinogens

Substance	Source
Carbon tetrachloride	Air pollution
Chloroform	Air pollution
Vinyl chloride	Air pollution and food
Asbestos	Occupational exposure
Radon	Pollution from soil or water below a home
Trihalomethanes	Drinking water
DDT (and, possibly, other pesticides)	Food
Cigarette smoke	Direct or second-hand exposure

As our environment exposes us to more and more carcinogens, we need to utilize dietary strategies to increase our defenses against free radicals and to avoid known carcinogens as much as possible. A cautious approach to anti-oxidant supplementation should be considered as an integral part of a well-formulated multiple vitamin and mineral preparation. This strategy is a practical, efficient, and convenient way to ensure more effective levels of these anti-cancer nutrients if the supplements are combined with the related nutritional advice of the Winning Weigh program.

The potential benefits of supplementation become even more impressive when you look at the health issues that pertain to calcium intake. A recent study concluded that the average woman in our society continues to ingest less than 500 mg of calcium per day. This low level of calcium intake persists in spite of the numerous health articles and general warnings recommending that women pay closer attention to increasing the amount of calcium in their diet. As noted earlier in this book, postmenopausal osteoporosis is a major health problem today. This is indeed unfortunate when you realize that it is a condition that is almost completely preventable through optimal calcium intake throughout a woman's lifetime. (Of course, physical activity and exercise improve bone mineral status, working synergistically with calcium.) A daily calcium intake of 800-1000 mg per day up until the menopausal years would greatly enhance bone mineral density and in turn minimize the risk of subsequent osteoporosis development.

The Western Electric Study has shown that calcium deficiency is not just a woman's issue. This Chicago study followed 1954 men for a 19-year period, examining dietary intake records for various nutrients. One of the main findings in the study was that men with the highest calcium intake (above 1200 mg per day) had a 75 percent lower chance of developing colon cancer. To appreciate the importance of this finding, you must realize that colon/rectal cancer is the second leading cause of cancer death in North America (after lung cancer). The incidence in men has increased 39 percent from 1930 to 1986. It will affect one in twenty people (5 percent of the population).

Calcium appears to reduce colon cancer risk through two mechanisms: it binds to bile acids, forming an insoluble calcium soap, thus preventing the conversion of bile acids to cancer-causing sterols in the large bowel; and it slows down the replication rate of cells that line the large bowel, an effect that is also associated with decreased cancer development.

To derive these benefits, men and women need to increase their calcium intake. Calcium supplementation in a dose of 500 mg per day would benefit most people.

Studies also suggest that improved calcium intake across the population would be likely to reduce the number of cases of high blood pressure in our society by its relaxing action on the muscular walls of arteries.

As vitamin D and calcium metabolism are intimately related, a multiple vitamin and mineral that includes 400 I.U. of vitamin D and 500 mg of calcium (preferably calcium citrate and/or calcium carbonate) would be sufficient supplementation for most individuals.

There is now growing support in the scientific community for the inclusion of a well-formulated multiple vitamin and mineral supplement in the daily diet. Exhibit 3–10 shows two traditional-type multiple vitamin and mineral supplements and two of the more recent, anti-oxidant-enriched versions that are becoming more commomplace in the market. If you choose to take a multiple vitamin and mineral supplement, be sure to take it with meals to ensure maximum absorption.

Exhibit 3-10
Multiple Vitamin and Mineral Supplement

This general comparison contrasts the more traditional type of multiple vitamin and mineral supplements with the new generation of anti-oxidant-enriched preparations.

Not all of the ingredients contained within these products have been listed.

Vitamin/Mineral	Traditional Formulations of Multivitamins		New Generation of Anti-oxidant-enriched Multiple Vitamin and Mineral Supplements	
	Centrum Forte® High Potency Multiple Vitamin-Multimineral Formula Lederle	Jamieson Natural Sources Mega Vim 75 ®	Vitox Dietary Supplement of Vitamins and Minerals ® Interior Design Nutritionals 7500 I.U. 12,500 I.U.	Multiple Choice The Ultimate One ® Nu-Life
Vitamin A	4000 I.U.	10,000 I.U.	300 I.U.	5000 I.U.
Beta-carotene	1000 I.U.	—	500 mg	15,000 I.U.
Vitamin E	30 I.U.	150 I.U.	500 mg	100 I.U.
Vitamin C	90 mg	250 mg	400 I.U.	150 mg
Calcium	175 mg	—	100 µg	125 mg
Vitamin D	400 I.U.	400 I.U.	100 µg	400 I.U.
Selenium	25 µg	10 µg	6 mg	50 µg
Chromiun	25 µg	10 µg	15 mg	50 µg
Iron	10 mg	4 mg	3 mg	10 mg
Zinc	15 mg	1.5 mg	3.4 mg	12 mg
Vitamin B_1	2.25 mg	75 mg	40 mg	25 mg
Vitamin B_2	2.6 mg	75 mg	4 mg	25 mg
Niacin	20 mg	75 mg	12 µg	100 mg
Vitamin B_6	3 mg	75 mg	0.4 mg	25 mg
Vitamin B_{12}	9 µg	75 mg	50 mg	100 µg
Folic Acid	0.4 mg	0.4 mg	300 µg	1 mg
Pantothenic acid	10 mg	75 mg	2 mg	50 mg
Biotin	45 µg	75 mg	5 mg	50 µg
Copper	2 mg	1 mg	200 mg	1 mg
Manganese	5 mg	0.61 mg		5 mg
Magnesium	100 mg	50 mg		75 mg

We both take supplements in the ranges discussed in this section. For us, the potential long-term benefits of a vitamin and mineral supplementation program far outweigh the risks. This decision is based on our individual medical and family histories and a review of recent relevant literature.

To arrive at your own decision, please discuss the possibility of vitamin and mineral supplementation with your family doctor. We have already stressed the importance of seeing your physician before beginning this program, but we feel that it is also important to specifically discuss the viability of supplementation with them.

We have specified here the amounts that we recommend as your maximum supplementation. Remember that ***more is not better***. If you choose to take less than these amounts, that is fine, but we strongly recommend that you do not exceed them.

Sample Meals for Seven Days

We feel that you should plan and choose your own meals. In this book, we want to give you recipes for personal change, not recipes for dinner. That's what the Winning Weigh is all about: taking control of your life and making your own decisions. It's up to you to use the information we gave you in the last chapter to help you choose wisely and prepare your food in a healthy way. You know the principles – now make the program your own.

That said, we want to do something for the people who have asked us to at least provide some help to get them started. So here is a list of some of our favorite dishes. We have provided references to cookbooks whose versions we particularly enjoy. Those books are

Ruthe Eshleman and Mary Winston, **The American Heart Association Cookbook.** 5th ed. New York: Times Books, 1991.

Jeanne Jones, **Cook It Light**. New York: Macmillan, Toronto: Collier Macmillan, 1987.

Judy Leach, **Fare For Friends**. Toronto: Key Porter, 1983

Terry Joyce Blonder, **For Goodness' Sake: An Eating Well Guide to Creative Low-Fat Cooking**. Charlotte, Vt: Camden House Publishing, 1990.

Marion Rombauer Becker, **Joy of Cooking**. Rev. ed. Indianapolis: Bobbs-Merril, 1975.

Jane Brody's Good Food Book: Living the High-Carbohydrate Way. New York: Norton, 1985.

Anne Lindsay, **The Lighthearted Cookbook: Recipes for Healthy Heart Cooking.** Toronto: Key Porter, 1988. (Published in co-operation with the Heart and Stroke Foundation of Canada.)

Anne Lindsay, **Lighthearted Everyday Cooking**. Toronto: Macmillan of Canada, 1991. (Published in co-operation with the Heart and Stroke Foundation of Canada.)

Martha Rose Shulman, ***Mediterranean Light: Delicious Recipes from the World's Healthiest Cuisine.*** New York: Bantam, 1989.

Julee Rosso and Sheila Lukins, ***The New Basics Cookbook.*** New York: Workman, 1989.

Anne Lindsay, ***Smart Cooking: Quick and Tasty Recipes for Healthy Living.*** Toronto: Macmillan of Canada, 1986. (Published in co-operation with the Canadian Cancer Society.)

You may be surprised at how many of your own favorite recipes you can adapt to fit the Winning Weigh program. Here are some of ours:

Chicken Dishes

1. Chicken Jerusalem - ***The American Heart Association Cookbook***
2. Chicken with Orange - ***The American Heart Association Cookbook***
3. Oriental Chicken Salad - ***Fare for Friends*** (Omit the almonds and sesame seeds.)
4. Orange Orange Roughy - ***The New Basics Cookbook***
5. Chicken Kiev - ***The New Basics Cookbook***
6. Chicken Jambalaya - ***Joy of Cooking*** (Do not use butter.)
7. Oriental Chicken and Noodles - ***The American Heart Association Cookbook***
8. Shredded Chicken with Green Peppers and Carrots - ***The American Heart Association Cookbook***
9. Oven-Barbequed Chicken - ***The American Heart Association Cookbook***
10. Spanish Chicken - ***The American Heart Association Cookbook***
11. Chicken Cacciatore with Noodles - ***Jane Brody's Good Food Book***
12. Chicken with Carrots and Cabbage - ***Jane Brody's Good Food Book***

Fish Dishes and Seafood
1. Poached Salmon in Rosé Wine - *Fare for Friends*
2. Grouper in Tomato Sauce - *Fare for Friends*
3. Fresh Cod à la Portuguese - *Joy of Cooking* (Omit butter swirl.)
4. Tomatoes Stuffed with Seafood - *Joy of Cooking* (Use skim or 1% milk.)
5. Fettucini with Mussel Sauce - *Jane Brody's Good Food Book*
6. Hearty Halibut - *The American Heart Association Cookbook*
7. Poached Fish - *The American Heart Association Cookbook*
8. Shrimp Gumbo - *The American Heart Association Cookbook*
9. Scallops Oriental - *The American Heart Association Cookbook*
10. Bean Sprout Tuna Chow Mein - *The American Heart Association Cookbook*
11. Flounder with Mexican Hot Sauce - *Jane Brody's Good Food Book*
12. Seafood Pilaf - *Jane Brody's Good Food Book*

Great Complex Carbohydrate Meals
1. Ratatouille - *Fare for Friends*
2. Vegetarian Chili - *Jane Brody's Good Food Book*
3. Vegetarian Shepherd's Pie - *Jane Brody's Good Food Book*
4. Chick-pea and Pasta Soup - *Jane Brody's Good Food Book*
5. Lentil Soup - *The American Heart Association Cookbook*
6. Baked Beans - *The American Heart Association Cookbook*
7. Scalloped Eggplant Italian - *The American Heart Association Cookbook*
8. Any Bean Salad - *The American Heart Association Cookbook*
9. Complementary Pizza - *The American Heart Association Cookbook*

10. Stuffed Peppers - ***The American Heart Association Cookbook***
11. Carrot and Broccoli Stir Fry - ***Jane Brody's Good Food Book***
12. The Best Ratatouille - ***Jane Brody's Good Food Book***

Appetizers
1. Marinated Tomato Salad - ***Fare for Friends*** (Use bocconcino cheese instead of feta cheese and omit dressing.)
2. Crunchy Lentil Salad - ***The New Basics Cookbook***
3. Basic Bruschetta - ***The New Basics Cookbook***

Low-Fat Dairy Meals
1. Zucchini Cheese Casserole - ***The American Heart Association Cookbook***
2. Breakfast Shake - ***Jane Brody's Good Food Book***
3. Cottage Cheese Toasties - ***Jane Brody's Good Food Book***

Side Dishes
1. Rosemary Potatoes - ***Fare for Friends***
2. Fresh Tomato Salsa - **The New Basics Cookbook** (This is an excellent dip for low-fat biscuits and crisp breads.)

Homemade Desserts and Breads
1. Apple-Ricotta Pie - ***Jane Brody's Good Food Book***
2. Apple Muffins - ***The American Heart Association Cookbook***
3. "Grate" Zucchini Bread - ***Jane Brody's Good Food Book***
4. Bran Bread - ***Fare for Friends***
5. Multi-Grain Bread - ***The New Basics Cookbook***

Seven Days on the Winning Weigh

Feel free to use our favorite recipes if they will help you get started. As you find your own health-promoting foods you can add to the list. Once you understand the principles of the Winning Weigh program, you can decide for yourself whether a particular recipe meets the requirements of a healthy diet.

To help you further, here is a sample seven-day menu made up of Winning Weigh meals. We are going to draw upon some of the recipes from the preceding list.

KEY
CC = Complex Carbohydrate
DP = Low-fat dairy protein
FP = Low-fat flesh protein
NCB = No-calorie beverage

DAY ONE

Breakfast — Fiber Points
Dairy Protein Meal
CC 1 pumpernickel bagel — 1.0
DP ricotta cheese (spread on bagel)
CC 1 grapefruit — 0.5
NCB black coffee

Snack
CC 1 apple — 1.0

Lunch
Complex Carbohydrate Meal
CC chicken noodle soup — 0.5
CC mixed chef's salad (oil and vinegar dressing) — 1.0
CC 2 slices plain, whole wheat bread — 2.0
NCB soda water

Dinner
Flesh Protein Meal
FP   Chicken with Orange
CC   1 baked potato with low-fat plain yogurt   1.5
CC   1/2 cup Any Bean Salad
      (with oil and vinegar dressing)   2.0
NCB diet drink

Snack
CC   1 banana   1.0

                        Total   10.5 pts

DAY TWO

Breakfast   **Fiber Points**
Dairy Protein Meal
DP   8-10 oz. low-fat yogurt
CC   slice one nectarine and add it to yogurt   1.0
CC   add 1/2 cup high-fiber cereal to yogurt   3.5
NCB herbal tea

Lunch
Complex Carbohydrate Meal
CC   Pasta with Tomato Sauce   1.0
CC   mixed green salad (oil and vinegar dressing)   1.0
CC   whole wheat roll   1.0
NCB mineral water

Snack
CC   2 plums   1.0

Dinner
Flesh Protein Meal
FP   Hearty Halibut   1.0

CC	1/2 cup brown rice (boiled)	2.0
CC	cranberry juice, diluted with water	

                                                               Total   11.5 pts

DAY THREE

Breakfast   **Fiber Points**

Complex Carbohydrate Meal

CC	1 pumpernickel bagel	1.0
CC	1 tbsp jam (spread on bagel)	1.0
CC	1 cup sliced cantaloupe	0.5
NCB	herbal tea	

Snack

CC	1 apple	1.0

Lunch

Flesh Protein Meal

FP	1 small tin salmon (water packed)	
CC	2 slices whole wheat bread	2.0
CC	1 sliced tomato	0.5
CC	1 bowl vegetable soup	1.0

Dinner

Dairy Protein Meal

DP	Vegetarian Lasagna with Ricotta Cheese	1.0
CC	mixed green salad	1.0
NCB	soda water	

Snack

CC	2 cups popcorn (no butter or salt)	1.0

                                                            Total   10.0 pts

DAY FOUR

Breakfast		**Fiber Points**
Complex Carbohydrate Meal		
CC	1 bowl hot oatmeal	2.5
CC	2 slices whole wheat toast	2.0
CC	jam	1.0
CC	diluted fruit juice	

Lunch		
Dairy Protein Meal		
DP	Zucchini Cheese Casserole	
CC	zucchini, onion, tomatoes	1.0
NCB	spring water	

Snack		
CC	two peaches	2.0

Dinner		
Flesh Protein Meal		
FP	Fettucine with Mussel Sauce	1.0
CC	fettucine	
CC	2 dinner rolls (plain)	1.0
CC	mixed green salad (oil and vinegar dressing)	1.0

Dessert		
CC	lemon sherbet	
NCB	black coffee	

Total   11.5 pts

DAY FIVE

Breakfast   **Fiber Points**
Dairy Protein Meal
DP   8-10 oz low-fat plain yogurt
CC   add 1/2 cup fresh fruit   1.0
CC   add 1/2 cup high-fiber cereal   3.5
CC   diluted fruit juice

Snack
CC   1 banana   1.0

Lunch
Complex Carbohydrate Meal
CC   Penne alla Arrabiate   1.0
CC   mixed green salad
     (oil and vinegar dressing)   1.0
CC   1 dinner roll   0.5
NCB mineral water

Snack
CC   1 apple   1.0

Dinner
Flesh Protein Meal
FP   Poached Salmon in Rosé Wine
CC   steamed rice   0.75
CC   cooked carrots   1.0
CC   1 slice whole wheat bread (plain)   1.0
NCB spring water

                                    Total   10.75 pts

DAY SIX

Breakfast	**Fiber Points**
Complex Carbohydrate Meal	
CC 2 low-fat bran muffins	4.0
CC diluted fruit juice	

Snack
CC 2 high-fiber biscuits	1.0
CC 1 nectarine	1.0

Lunch
Dairy Protein Meal
DP compressed cottage cheese on a	
CC pumpernickel bagel	1.0
CC large fruit salad	2.0
NCB black coffee	

Dinner
Flesh Protein Meal
FP Chicken Jerusalem	1.0
CC mushrooms, artichoke hearts, tomatoes	2.0
NCB mineral water	

Snack
CC large bowl popcorn (no butter or salt)	2.0
Total	**14.0 pts**

DAY SEVEN

Breakfast   Fiber Points
Dairy Protein Meal
DP 3 oz partly-skimmed mozzarella cheese
CC melted over an open-faced bagel   1.0
CC 1 grapefruit   0.5
NCB herbal tea

Lunch
Flesh Protein Meal
FP sliced turkey breast
CC 2 slices whole wheat bread   2.0
CC tomatoes, lettuce   1.0
CC 1 bowl vegetable soup   1.0
NCB mineral water

Snack
CC 2 plums   1.0

Dinner
Complex Carbohydrate meal
CC Ratatouille (onions, green pepper, tomatoes,
   eggplant, zucchini)   1.0
CC boiled rice (1/2 cup)   2.0
CC fruit salad (2 cups)   2.0
NCB diet drink   2.0

            Total **10.5 pts**

People Who Are Lactose- or Dairy-Intolerant

A significant number of adults are unable to digest milk sugars (lactose) properly or are sensitive to dairy proteins. The two-staple system can be easily adapted to the needs of those who are lactose- or dairy-intolerant. If this is the case for you, you should try applying the following modifications of the Winning Weigh program.

1. Have a complex carbohydrate meal for breakfast each day.

2. 3 or 4 times a week, have a flesh protein meal for lunch and another for dinner.

3. On the other days of the week, have a flesh protein meal for lunch or dinner, but make your third meal another complex-carbohydrate meal.

4. Consider taking a calcium supplement (500 mg), as well as a multiple vitamin that contains 400 I.U. of vitamin D.

5. You can substitute soybean products like tofu in place of yogurt or cheese in dairy protein meals. Egg white, which has a different protein than milk products and contains no lactose, can also be used as a main ingredient of a dairy protein meal. Try an egg white omelet, you'll be pleasantly surprised.

6. Wherever possible, choose complex-carbohydrates that are high in calcium. Some of the foods that will help you compensate for the lack of dairy products are beans, artichokes, broccoli, beet greens, collards, dandelion greens, kale, mustard greens, spinach, Swiss chard, turnip greens, leeks, okra, rutabagas, and rhubarb. Tofu and canned sardines or salmon (with bones) are also relatively good sources of calcium.

Starting Right Now . . .

1. Think of your body as a laboratory experiment. Keep working with this image for at least 30 days. Determine what quantities of food satisfy your hunger. If you find that your weight goes up or you are feeling full on less food than you normally eat, then adjust the quantities accordingly.

2. Experiment with gradually cutting back quantities. You will probably find you can easily adjust to smaller portions over a span of a few weeks. Remember how flexible your silent partner is.

3. Buy or borrow a few of the cookbooks we've listed or ones *you* enjoy. Begin to cut out recipes from newspapers and magazines or exchange them with friends. Experiment with adapting them to fit the Winning Weigh program.

4. Get a group of friends interested in joining your wellness journey by throwing a potluck dinner. You can each bring one item that is in keeping with the advice given in **The Winning Weigh.**

5. Remember that each day is a new beginning for you....Enjoy!

Exercise

Being active is one of the great joys of living. In earlier times, hunting and gathering food was a basic part of human existence. Exercise was not some isolated activity, carefully scheduled three times a week, but a necessary part of surviving. Times have changed. With conveniences such as cars and elevators, our activity level has dropped dramatically. Many people have desk jobs; exercise is no longer an automatic component of our lifestyle. If you are not very active, we want to help you rediscover the pleasure of being mobile.

We can't design one exercise program that would suit everyone on the Winning Weigh program. Everyone is unique, with different levels of fitness and health. It is up to *you* to set your long-term goals and then decide how much time and effort you are willing to invest in this quest for a more healthy life.

We *will* offer you three different exercise programs that you can adapt for your own goals, needs, and circumstances: the Power Walker – a light activity program for people who hate to exercise; the Wellness-Oriented Exerciser – an aerobic program for people who want the benefits of aerobic exercise; and the Elite Endurance Athlete – a nutritional program for dedicated athletes. Whatever program you choose, it will help you toward your overall wellness goals.

For many people, the Power Walker program may prove too much too early. Be realistic and invoke your compassionate commitment. If you are seriously out of shape and are not ready for a three-mile walk, start on a more leisurely, recreational level. The first step up from the basement may be simply walking to and from the subway or bus, or getting off the bus early to walk part way to work. A thousand-mile journey begins with one small step. Keep this saying in mind as you walk that initial block, cover that flight of stairs, or swim for five minutes on your back. Have compassion for where you are at this very moment! Gradually build up to walking for 30 minutes,

Exhibit 3–11
Choosing the Right Program

Use the following descriptions to choose the program that suits you.

The Power Walker
- You hate to exercise.
- You have medical problems that prevent you from getting aerobic exercise.
- You are badly out of shape.

The Wellness-Oriented Exerciser
- You are willing to exercise aerobically for at least 20 minutes, three times a week.
- You want the benefits of accelerated weight reduction, energy gain, and cardiovascular health.
- You have followed the Power Walker program for a while and are ready to move up to the next level.

The Elite Endurance Athlete
- You are already in top aerobic condition.
- Fitness and training dominate much of your leisure time and you participate in marathon tests of endurance.
- You want nutritional and training advice to enhance your athletic performance.

five to seven times each week. Most people can manage this amount of exercise on a daily basis. Begin looking for more challenging ways to get your body in motion. Try to see your daily activities as opportunities to exercise. Why not leave your car at the *far* end of the parking mall? Whatever you decide – start now.

Try walking at a brisk pace and focusing on swinging your arms as you go about your daily routine. Very soon you'll find yourself at a new level of fitness. You'll then want to choose a more vigorous form of exercise. You might want to consider cycling, jogging, or using an aerobic gym machine. Most gyms have stationary bikes, stair climbers, treadmills, and rowing machines.

Enjoy the benefits of small changes. Get rid of that all-or-nothing attitude and slowly adapt one of the Winning Weigh exercise programs into your life. Even if you can only walk four miles (6.5 km) a week, that is a beginning. You *will* experience a benefit from this commitment.

The Light Activity Program: The Power Walker

By burning as few as 2000 calories per week, you will begin to notice the benefits of light activity. Burning these calories is important for your well-being whether or not you want to lose weight. How can you burn off 2000 calories? By walking one kilometre, you burn as many calories as you weigh in kilograms. So if you weigh 70 kg, you would burn 70 calories by walking a kilometre. Let's say you walk five kilometres (three miles) a day, six times a week. Now figure out how many calories that would burn:

70 calories x 5 km x 6 times per week = 2100 calories

So a three-mile (5 km) walk, six times a week, is just enough physical activity to significantly decrease your risks of heart disease and certain cancers.

If you wish, you can jog some of those kilometers instead of walking them. The main difference, however, between walking a mile and jogging a mile is how fast you get across the finish line. You burn the same number of calories either way. Jogging will provide some additional aerobic benefits, but walking is a tremendously underrated method of exercise: you burn the same number of calories as you do jogging; you can do it almost anywhere; and you don't need any fancy equipment.

Swimming is not quite as effective a method of burning calories for people who are overweight. Fat makes you more buoyant in the water, which means you sink less. The higher you sit in the water, the less force you need to move through it. Therefore, a heavier person uses *less* energy to swim a mile than a lean person. Jazz dancing and ballroom dancing are good supplements to the Power Walker program. One hour of dancing is roughly equivalent to a three-mile walk.

Wear a proper pair of shoes for your power walk, preferably jogging shoes. Choose different routes to keep your walks interesting. Listen to your favorite music as you walk to help maintain your pace and make your exercising more enjoyable. Vary it sometimes by taping a talk show or planning a letter while you walk.

To burn more calories during your power walk, you can carry one-pound hand weights or wrist weights. By swinging your arms briskly as you walk, you will further increase your heart rate, making the power walk more of an aerobic workout.

Eventually, you will probably find the power walk is not enough of a challenge. This means you're getting into shape. Try alternating walking and jogging. Jog until you feel tired, then walk until you recover. Don't be surprised when one day you find yourself able to jog the entire distance.

The Wellness-Oriented Exerciser

To benefit from aerobic exercise, you must get your heart beating within your aerobic training heart-rate zone. This zone is between 60 and 85 percent of your maximum attainable heart rate. Your maximum attainable heart rate is how fast your heart would beat if you were to exercise all-out to the point of complete exhaustion. Fortunately, you don't actually have to reach this point. You can estimate your maximum attainable heart rate by subtracting your present age from 220:

Maximum attainable heart rate = 220 minus your age

Low end of aerobic heart-rate zone = heart rate x 0.6

High end of aerobic heart-rate zone = heart rate x 0.85

Let's look at an example. If you are 40 years old, your maximum attainable heart rate is 180 beats per minute (220 – 40). Your aerobic heart-rate zone ranges from 108 beats per minute (180 x 0.6) to 153 beats per minute (180 x 0.85), so you can attain the benefits of aerobic exercise by keeping your heart beating between 108 and 153 beats per minute for 20 to 45 minutes, at least three times per week.

Exercising at 60 percent of your maximum attainable rate is so comfortable that you could maintain a conversation without getting winded. Unknowingly, most people jog at a pace that puts their heart rate between 70 and 75 percent of their maximum attainable rate. If you are just starting with aerobic exercise, you should aim for about 65 percent of your maximum attainable rate. If you are already in good shape, aim for about 75 percent. There is really no reason to push yourself any harder than this.

Actually, it is better to slow down your aerobic exercise and cover a longer distance (or spend a longer time doing it), than to push yourself too hard and finish sooner. In terms of weight loss, you burn more fat working at 60 to 70 percent of your maximum attainable heart rate than you do by working at a more intense rate. Your body requires oxygen to burn fat. When you are working at a higher intensity, your body cannot deliver enough oxygen to satisfy your muscles completely. Therefore, your muscles generate more energy by burning carbohydrates rather than fat. So if you are trying to burn extra body fat, slow down and spend a little more time exercising. Aim for 45 minutes per exercise session.

You will be amazed at how quickly your body adapts, once you initiate an aerobic program. We have seen a great many people who were extremely overweight or out of shape achieve fantastic results in short periods of time. We have seen first-time joggers, who originally required an average ten or eleven minutes to complete a mile, improve their times to eight, seven, or even an elite six minutes per mile.

This improvement results from an increase in the muscles' oxygen consumption and the number of sites within the body that can generate energy. With more available energy, the muscles can do more work, enabling you to run faster (or row harder or whatever).

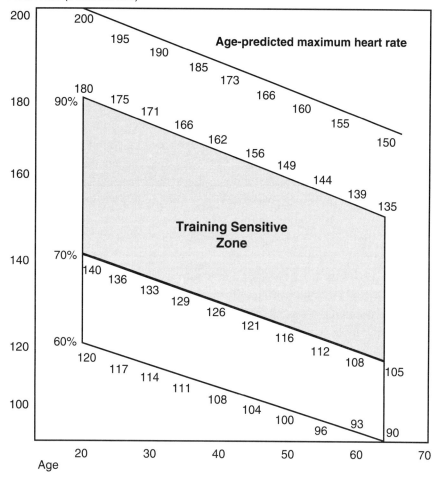

Maximal heart rates and training sensitive zones for use in aerobic training programs for people of different ages. The zone between 60 - 70% of your maximum heart rate is sufficient to derive aerobic benefits and at the same time is not so demanding as to produce significant discomfort.

Your overall exercise performance will gradually improve as a result of regular participation. You don't have to overexert yourself. Your speed, endurance, and strength will improve as a natural response to the aerobic exercise itself. Studies show that in six to eight weeks you can improve your oxygen intake capacity by *15 to 25 percent.*

Types of Aerobic Exercise

Any activity that keeps your heart beating within your aerobic training heart-rate zone is good aerobic exercise. It doesn't matter what you do – jogging, cycling, rowing, running up and down the stairs – anything that keeps your heart pumping fast. When the weather is bad, and you can't go out for your run, there are many popular alternatives. Stationary bikes, rowing machines, cross-country machines, treadmills, mini-trampolines, stair climbers, and swimming pools are available all year round.

In terms of calories burned, four miles of outdoor biking is equivalent to one mile of walking or jogging. This exercise is only aerobic, however, if your legs are in constant motion. The minute you start coasting, your heart rate will drop below the aerobic training zone. Keeping up this pace on city streets is usually impossible.

Aerobic classes, ironically, are not always an effective form of aerobic exercise. Most of the classes do not maintain your heart rate within the aerobic heart-rate zone for more than 20 minutes. Many are aimed primarily at muscle-toning and flexibility. They are great as an overall conditioner, but you should still jog at least two miles after each class or get at least 20 minutes of aerobic exercise during the class.

To begin, commit yourself to an aerobic program just for eight weeks. You'll probably find you like it.

If you have not exercised for a long time, consult your doctor before embarking on an ambitious aerobic program. Begin with 20-minute exercise sessions and gradually work up to 45 minutes. A 45-minute session maximizes the amount of fat you will continue to burn after exercising.

To cash in on the major aerobic benefits of jogging, you should cover at least 15 miles (24 km) per week. If you jog more than 25 miles (40 km) per week, however, you may develop shin splints, ankle problems, or knee problems. Jogging these long distances causes excessive wear and tear on your joints. As in most things, moderation is the key to long-term success.

Measure other forms of aerobic exercise, such as swimming and working out on stationary bikes, rowing machines, cross-country machines, treadmills, mini-trampolines, and stair climbers, by the length of time you spend on them, not by the "distance" you cover. All that matters is the length of time that your heart rate stays within your aerobic training heart-rate zone.

If you are training three days a week, these days should not be consecutive. You need to train every second day to sustain the training effect.

Don't push yourself to exhaustion. Make exercise something you enjoy. This precaution doesn't mean, however, that you shouldn't give yourself a bit of a challenge. Pushing yourself a little will add exhilaration to your exercise pattern.

The Elite Athlete

If you are a competitive athlete, you probably don't need our advice on training techniques. We can, however, point out a few Winning Weigh nutrition tips that will give you an edge over the competition. To begin with, it is especially important for you to eat a diet high in complex carbohydrates. The Winning Weigh nutritional program is a perfect way to load yourself with carbohydrates every day. Eat the complex-carbohydrate-only meal three to four hours prior to your daily workout. This will load your liver's carbohydrate fuel tank and help prevent hypoglycemic symptoms from appearing during your workout.

During aerobic exercise, up to 10 percent of your energy comes from the breakdown of muscle tissue protein. Therefore, it is wise to have some protein after your exercise to prevent breakdown of your muscle tissue. An hour after your workout, eat either your low-fat flesh or low-fat dairy protein meal. Remember, both of these meals also contain a substantial amount of complex carbohydrates, which will reload the stores of carbohydrates in your liver and muscles.

About 20 to 30 minutes before your workout, you should drink 13 to 20 ounces of water. You should also drink 8 to 10 ounces of water every 15 minutes during a prolonged training session or competitive marathon race. This helps prevent overheating and dehydration during exercise. Like the water in your car's radiator, the water in your bloodstream transports the heat generated from your exercising muscles to the surface of your body, where it escapes, primarily through sweat. You lose between one and three quarts of water per hour during exercise, so dehydration can occur quite easily. Losing 3 to 4 percent of your water volume through perspiration can decrease endurance performance by up to 30 percent. Further water loss can result in serious dehydration or even heat stroke. Incidentally, as well as being more refreshing, cold water (5°C, or 40° F) is absorbed into the bloodstream much faster and more efficiently than water at room temperature.

Profuse sweating also results in the loss of electrolytes and minerals. You should take approximately one gram of salt for every quart of water you drink during exercise to prevent a life-threatening condition know as **hyponatremia** (very low concentration of sodium in the blood).

When your aerobic exercise session ends for the day, replace the fluids in your body just beyond the point of satisfying your thirst. Thirst is a reasonably good indicator of your fluid needs, but by the time you get thirsty during exercise, your blood volume is already down by about one quart of water. In other words, you are already approaching dehydration. So remember: drink before, during, and after exercise.

The best drink to have after exercise is one part of any juice and three parts cold soda water. The juice will provide carbohydrates to restore your blood sugar quickly and will also provide potassium to replace what you lost in perspiration. The soda water will re-establish the proper balance of water and electrolytes in your bloodstream.

Some recent research indicates that athletes use vitamins B_2 and B_6 faster than other people. Both of these vitamins are necessary for energy production. Aerobic athletes may also be more likely to sustain oxygen damage to their muscles during exercise. Studies indicate that much of this tissue damage can be minimized by supplementing vitamin E, vitamin C, and beta-carotene in doses of 200-400 I.U., 500-1,000 mg, and 10,000-20,000 I.U., respectively. Therefore, it is advisable that aerobic athletes take a multiple vitamin and mineral tablet to supplement the Winning Weigh nutritional program. Be sure that the multiple vitamin tablet you choose contains no more than 7,500 I.U. of vitamin A to prevent the risk of toxicity.

There is no question that good nutrition and fluid replacement have a major impact on athletic performance. Use the Winning Weigh nutritional program to complement your aerobic-endurance training – capitalize on the Winning Weigh's competitive edge.

Long-Term Compliance

Despite the fantastic benefits of aerobic exercise, you may still see exercising as an unpleasant and uncomfortable chore. If so, you need to learn how to make it fun! Exercising should give you the same feeling of rejuvenation and revitalization as dancing to your favorite music does. In fact, we strongly recommend that you listen to your favorite music while you perform aerobic exercise. Listening to upbeat songs will make continuous movement feel natural. Jazz dancing and aerobic dance classes, which are always accompanied by music, are great forms of aerobic exercise.

When you first start an exercise program, you will probably have to take firm charge of your body. If you haven't been exercising regularly, your body will be weak, tired, and addicted to the foods and behaviors that kept you out of shape. Listening to your body at this point won't do you any good. It will dictate terms that would keep you fat or out of shape. As Newton so aptly stated, "A body at rest stays at rest." You must, therefore, write down a fitness goal and decide how you're going to fit exercise into your schedule. What would work best for you? A morning walk? An evening jog? Perhaps a workout at lunchtime? Make your exercise times convenient, so that you will be more inclined to stick to them.

If your body is still reluctant, then it's up to your mind to force it into action. Exercise even when you don't feel like it. If you can get your body into action at times like these, in a matter of minutes both your body and mind will both feel better. We guarantee it!

Some people start their exercise programs believing that exercise hurts or is unpleasant. Don't equate mild discomfort at the beginning of a program with the way you feel about exercise itself. Go beyond the superficial; look deeper and ask yourself how you *really* feel, knowing that you are improving your wellness through exercise. You will probably begin to realize the power and control you can gain over your life by adhering to a regular program of exercise. Instinctively, you know it is the right thing to do for *you.* And once the exercise program becomes a part of your life, the unpleasantness will only be a memory.

Improved psychological well-being is one of the major benefits of exercise. Take advantage of the runner's high, that pleasurable feeling that kicks in 20 to 30 minutes into an aerobic workout. View your aerobic time as wellness time – time to clear your head, move your body, and get a physical and psychological lift. Enjoy the moment. Try to see exercise as an opportunity to recharge your battery.

Physical activity *can* change your mood. Learn to anticipate the positive feeling of well-being that comes from exercising. Don't let glum days, down days, depressing days, or boring days get you down. Exercise is a good way to leave those self-destructive emotions behind and to get on with the happy, positive life you deserve.

If you're still not convinced about the positive, uplifting benefits provided by aerobic exercise, then we challenge you to take the Winning Weigh Mood Test, provided in Exhibit 3–12.

Exhibit 3-12
The Winning Weigh Mood Test

1. Choose a day on which you should really exercise, but you feel too lethargic or low-spirited.

2. Rate your mood on a scale of one to ten. One signifies total depression. For absolute elation, score a 10 (lucky you!).

3. Follow through with your aerobic exercise program, even though you don't feel like doing it.

4. Now rate your mood again. If you have been honest with yourself, we are positive that your score will be substantially higher than before you exercised.

Sometimes you will encounter a stumbling block not before you exercise, but ***during*** the activity itself. This is where you will find the principles of in-the-moment choices are most obvious. Jim and I have often been out for a run together, feeling anxious about the distance or the pace, wondering if we would ever finish. Most of this nervous feeling comes from looking beyond the challenge of this very moment. By focusing on what lies ahead, you feel nothing but the seemingly impossible weight of your goal and, consequently, lose the pleasure of the present.

While training for a marathon, I habitually found myself anxious at the 12-mile mark of a 20-mile run. I tried visualizing myself calmly jogging, settling in to appreciate the beauty of the park I was running through. It worked. Instead of being anxious about the future, I fully enjoyed the present moment. You, too, will learn how to create a calming visualization for yourself in the section entitled Adopting a Winning Attitude.

Remember to never to push yourself to exhaustion. A patient of ours who started out overweight and out of shape now runs marathons a few times a year. He says that when he jogs, he concentrates on the idea of conserving his energy. He intentionally never pushes himself to the point of pain or exhaustion because he knows that he will have a negative reaction, both physically and psychologically. "I want to wake up tomorrow and look forward to my exercise session. I don't want to dread it," he says. If you push yourself too hard, it makes sense that you would be tired and resentful about exercising the next time. And your psychological outlook and day-to-day energy have everything to do with staying on track.

Pushing yourself too hard is detrimental to your health and well-being, but there is nothing wrong with challenging yourself a little bit. You'll feel good about yourself if you follow through. Remaining faithful to an aerobic exercise requires perseverance and dedication. Vince Lombardi said, "I never knew a man worth his salt who deep down in his heart did not appreciate the grind and discipline necessary to become a champion." The inner feeling of success and achievement remains long after the mild discomfort of exercise ends.

How do you know you won't enjoy a regular aerobic exercise program if you don't try it? Give yourself a chance to experience the physical and mental benefits. Decide ***now*** to stick with an aerobic program for at least eight consecutive weeks. We're sure that it will become a positive and permanent feature in your life. You will come to rely on it as a source of rejuvenation.

Starting Right Now . . .

Choose the exercise program that is right for you: the Power Walker, the Wellness-Oriented Exerciser, the Elite Endurance Athlete, or one you have devised for yourself.

Visit your doctor before starting a demanding program. Find out whether she or he recommends a stress test, electrocardiogram, or other test before you commit to an exercise routine.

If you have flu-like symptoms or diarrhea accompanied by a fever, do not exercise until you have been well for a week.

Now – go for it!

Summary

Exercise is an important part of healthy living. You should be working on a program that is appropriate for you.

1. The Power Walker
Burning 2000 calories will improve your health and lower your risks of heart disease and certain cancers. For most of us, this can be done by walking about three miles (5 km) each day. Jogging and dancing are good substitutes for walking. Cycling and swimming can also provide benefits.

2. The Wellness-Oriented Exerciser
Aerobic exercise will improve your body's ability to use oxygen, improve your cardiovascular system, and burn off unwanted fat. You should have 20- to 45-minute sessions three times per week.

3. The Elite Endurance Athlete
Eat your complex-carbohydrate-only meal three to four hours before you work out. Eat one of your protein meals an hour after you work out. Drink 13 to 20 ounces of cold water 30 minutes before you start to exercise. Continue to drink 8 to 10 ounces of water every 15 minutes during a long exercise session or competitive marathon. After exercising, drink a glass of one part juice and three parts soda water. Keep drinking even after you are no longer thirsty. Consider taking a multi-vitamin to ensure you get enough vitamin B2, vitamin B6, vitamin E, vitamin C, and beta-carotene.

Looking Ahead . . .

By now you are familiar with the Winning Weigh's two-staple system. You can now use this nutritional information to help create a motivating force in your life. In Step 4, to further strengthen your motivation, we will help you discover the ***benefits*** of this knowledge through the process of setting your goals.

STEP 4   SETTING YOUR GOALS

The Winning Weigh's two-staple system, which you learned to apply in Step 3, is our solution to the many diversified nutritional facts available today. The system was designed to help you make wellness-oriented food and exercise choices. Now we are going to help you discover and define your own personal wellness goals. We know from experience that the goal-setting procedure will be a powerful tool for you. It will be your next step forward, one more move toward long-term success. It's your chance to plan exactly how to become the new, improved you.

You probably began reading ***The Winning Weigh*** in the first place because you had some personal goal in mind. You realized that there was something you stood to gain by reading this book. Now you need to build on that personal goal and make it the motivation for ***wellness changes*** in your life. We want to help you clarify what you are after and motivate you to succeed. Setting goals will make it easier for you to eat health-promoting foods and to stick to a program of regular exercise.

We recommend that you set your goals in a three-part exercise. In the first part, decide what you are now doing wrong or what you need to improve. In the second part, define how you intend to change your approach. In the third part, identify the benefits that the new approach would bring to your life.

All three parts are important, but the third part is the one that will push you to make long-term changes. The benefits you stand to gain will help you decide if the effort required to make the changes is really worth it to you. Only you can make that decision.

How Motivated Are You?

Are you happy with the way your body has responded to your past and present eating and exercise patterns? ***Try testing your motivation to make a commitment to change by filling out Exhibit 4–1 and answering the seven questions that follow.***

Exhibit 4–1

Are you happy with ...

Wellness Parameters	No	Yes	Yes, but I would like to improve
1. your present weight?			
2. your body shape?			
3. your fitness level?			
4. your blood cholesterol level?			
5. your blood pressure?			

If you are not completely happy about the *wellness parameters* listed in Exhibit 4–1, try writing a statement describing how you would rather be. We have provided a place for you to do that in the Wellness Planner, page 314. This statement is your mission statement, your goal for change. How would your life be improved if you reached the state described in your mission statement?
To help focus yourself, answer the following questions.

1. Would you feel better about yourself?   Yes   No
2. Would taking good care of your body make you feel more whole as a person?   Yes   No
3. Would looking better and feeling better about yourself make you more confident and enhance any of the following aspects of your life:

your career?	Yes	No
your family life?	Yes	No
your social life?	Yes	No
your sex life?	Yes	No

4. If you changed your habits, would that influence other people who are important to you to improve their dietary and exercise habits?
   Yes   No
5. Would it make you feel good to be a role model for these people?
   Yes   No
6. Are you personally motivated right now to live as long as you can with the highest degree of energy, quality, and passion?
   Yes   No

7. On a scale of 1 to 10 how motivated are you to set wellness goals for yourself? (Circle one.)

1	2	3	4	5	6	7	8	9	10
low level				motivation				high level	

Now, let's stop for a moment and see what has happened. If you answered "yes" to most of these questions, then you have become aware of the fact that you will probably feel better about yourself if you look good on the outside and are less prone to heart attacks and cancer on the inside.

Feeling good about yourself allows you to succeed. How you feel strongly determines how you behave or what you will automatically do. Changing how you feel about things is fundamental to changing how you behave in the long run.

How does this apply to wellness? Many times we see patients who only try to change how they behave without first becoming connected on an emotional level to what these behavioral changes represent to them. Generally speaking, these are people who go on diets in a desperate effort to lose weight. On a conscious level they tell themselves:

"Eat dull, tasteless carrot sticks – instead of orgasmic, premium double-fudge ice cream."

"Eat bland and boring cottage cheese for lunch – instead of a delicious deluxe hamburger."

"Ride a stationary bike – even though I hate the pain and it's the most uninspiring thing I've ever done."

These people are acting from a base of incongruency; that is, they are struggling to force themselves to do something when they would rather be doing something else that would provide them with more immediate pleasure. This approach to weight loss fails almost every time, if you look at long-term results. Real lasting change can only occur once your feeling about what you are doing and the action of doing it are congruent. With respect to nutrition and exercise, congruency means feeling good about acting in a health-promoting way rather than feeling deprived or punished. This feeling will only come from recognition of and enthusiasm for the benefits that the health-promoting behavior can provide for you.

You are already making decisions of this sort. You wouldn't use cocaine even though you have heard that it might provide a temporary pleasurable feeling. You know the consequences just aren't worth the momentary high. You need to apply the same kind of thinking to food. As long as you associate enjoyment with eating cheese cake instead of thinking about the potential damage from heart disease and cancer, you are setting yourself up for an ongoing internal conflict.

If you develop the right attitude, eating well and exercising will become easy. If you try to act without changing your attitude, you will always struggle to make it work. You need to *feel* that eating chicken with broccoli represents a more favorable outcome than eating a cheeseburger with French fries.

How motivated are you to take action to protect yourself from a terminal disease or major illness? Find out by answering the following questions:

1. Beginning at age 35 for men and age 45 for women, the chances of dying from coronary artery disease (caused by a buildup of cholesterol in the arteries of the heart) increases progressively and dramatically. According to many researchers there is unquestioned evidence that coronary artery disease is preventable in an overwhelming number of cases by dietary and lifestyle changes. What would it mean to your life, your future plans, and your happiness if you suffered a non-fatal but major heart attack within the next few years? Would the consequences to your life have

a devastating impact?
a moderate impact?
a mild impact?
no impact?

2. On a scale of 1 to 10 how motivated are you right now to begin eating better and exercising appropriately in order to defend against this disease? (Circle one.)

1	2	3	4	5	6	7	8	9	10
low level				motivation				high level	

3. What would it mean to your life, if you suffered a stroke in the next year and were left paralyzed on one side of your body? Would the consequences to your life have

    a devastating impact?
    a moderate impact?
    a mild impact?
    no impact?

4. On a scale of 1 to 10, how motivated are you right now to begin eating better and exercising appropriately in order to defend against this outcome? (Circle one.)

1	2	3	4	5	6	7	8	9	10
low level				motivation				high level	

5. (for women) Geneticists tell us that a minority of women who develop breast cancer are prone to this condition from genetic inheritance. A significant percentage of the cases of breast cancer are encouraged by environmental factors, including dietary practices and lack of physical activity. One in nine North American women will develop this deadly, terrible disease. In 1960, the ratio was one in twenty. So things are getting worse and will probably continue to do so as the population ages. What would it mean to your life, your future plans, and your happiness if you developed this disease within the next year? Would it create

    a devastating impact?
    a moderate impact?
    a mild impact?
    no impact?

6. On a scale of 1 to 10, how motivated are you right now to make the necessary dietary changes and develop the exercise habits needed to defend against this disease? (Circle one.)

1   2   3   4   5   6   7   8   9   10
low level   motivation   high level

7. Cancer of the colon and rectum is the second most common major cancer in North America. The incidence has increased 39 percent in the male population since 1930. Beginning at age 40, the risk for an individual begins to increase progressively and dramatically. One in every twenty persons becomes affected and the survival rate is only 50 percent as it stands today. Everyone agrees that better nutritional practices, better exercise habits, and early screening procedures would change the tide of this disease significantly. What would it mean to your life, your future plans, and your happiness if you developed this disease in the next year? Would it have

    a devastating impact?
    a moderate impact?
    a mild impact?
    no impact?

8. How motivated are you right now to begin eating better and exercising appropriately in order to defend against this disease?

1   2   3   4   5   6   7   8   9   10
low level   motivation   high level

We're sure you get the point. No one wants to develop any of these problems, yet most people are not taking the action required to protect themselves. One reason for that is that most of the time we don't pay attention to what is important in the long run because we get caught up in what seems to be urgent or more compelling in the moment. Life is full of distractions from our long-term goals. Every day you have to deal with your financial affairs. You may have business pressures pulling at you. You may have to drop the kids off or pick them up from the day care center or school. You need to find time for laundry, meetings, family commitments, social activities, shopping, lunch, housecleaning, car and appliance repairs, gardening, and any number of other obligations and deadlines. With all of these matters to deal with, you still need to find time to focus on your health. Other people with similar pressures, time restraints, and obligations are succeeding with a wellness-oriented diet and exercise program; you need to realize how important your health is to you and ***make wellness a priority for yourself.*** Now is the time to identify what changes you need to make in your approach to wellness.

Just sit back for a moment and close your eyes. Now, envision a realistic image of the healthiest, fittest, most vibrant person you could be if you followed through with the Winning Weigh program. Connect with this image by experiencing the power and energy that you would achieve in this state.

To determine your Wellness Image Goal, fill out the following Goal-Setting Questionnaire:

1. What body weight are you working to achieve? Give yourself a weight range that you feel you could maintain during the best and worst times.

   Target weight _____
   Range: Upper Limit _____Lower Limit _____

2. What physical activity or aerobic workout are you committed to starting right now?
   Type of activity_____
   _____

   (Examples: power walking, jogging, using a stair climber, stationary bicycle, or treadmill)
   Time or distance _____
   Frequency_____
   (number of workouts per week)

3. What would you like to work up to in the next six months?

   Type of activity_____
   Time or Distance_____
   Frequency_____

Wellness Foods

How do you plan to incorporate more wellness foods into your daily intake? List the foods you now want to focus on to enhance your health:

A. Complex Carbohydrates

B. Dietary Fiber

Which fiber-rich foods would you like to begin utilizing to attain 8 to 15 fiber points per day? Use the Fiber Scoreboard on page 293 to help you set your objectives.

Cholesterol Crunchers					Colon Cleaners

C. Fish

To cut down on your red meat, pork, and prepared meats intake, which fish will you focus on and how will you incorporate them into your diet? (e.g., lunch = water packed salmon from the tin, with tomato and lettuce on whole wheat bread or a bagel)

D. Protective foods
Which foods are you committed to consuming more regularly in order to decrease your cancer risk?

Foods high in beta-carotene:

Foods high in vitamin C:

Cruciferous vegetables:

Supplements:

Disease-Promoting Foods
What disease-promoting foods are you committed to minimizing or avoiding altogether? Let's look at your present eating habits, so you can see what you may need to change.

A. Saturated fats
Under the following headings, write down the foods that you tend to eat regularly (more than once a month).
  Red meat:

  Prepared meats (luncheon meats, cold cuts, and fast foods):

  Organ meats:

  Pork:

High-fat products (e.g., ice cream, sour cream, butter):

Pastries and baked goods:

B. Refined sugars
Added white sugar (e.g., in your coffee):

Candy:

Syrup:

C. Caffeine
What is the maximum amount per day that you are working toward? (e.g., 2 cups of coffee per day.)

D. Alcohol
What is the maximum number of drinks per week that you are intending to allow yourself? How much will you have to reduce your present consumption?
    1 drink = 1 beer
            1 - 8-oz. glass of wine
            1 oz. of hard liquor
Go back and put a check mark beside foods that you will commit to minimizing or avoiding altogether.

The Power of a Contract

Now, congratulate yourself! You have just entered a new realm of commitment and opportunity. The simple act of writing out your goals and intentions under the preceding headings has initiated some powerful changes. First of all, writing your goals down tremendously increases your probability of success. It's the difference between **wanting** to do something and actually **signing a contract** with yourself to make it happen. It's the moment in which you declare:

> This is what I now stand for; this is what I am committed to achieving!

Clarifying your goals strengthens your belief in yourself, and your capabilities. The goals you have just outlined for yourself are a concrete plan for incorporating the principles of **The Winning Weigh** into your life. You can now see how your plan will fit into the other dimensions of your life. Your wellness goals must become a part of your everyday existence. These goals will serve as a point of reference that you can access each day to help you stay on track.

Time, Experience, and Repetition

The third part of setting goals is to understand how they will serve you as time passes. The only way to change your approach permanently and develop new long-term health-promoting habits is to align your feelings with your actions. By finding this congruency, you can minimize the internal struggles you face. The less you need to struggle, the less likely you are to lose.

This alignment may be difficult at first, simply because you have not programmed yourself over your lifetime to eat foods that are good for you or to find the time to work out regularly. Be patient; it may be a while before you are consistently congruent in your new wellness behavior. It takes time to develop new habits and to shed old, destructive ones. To help you develop a healthy addiction to good food and exercise, you must read your goals every day for the next ten weeks. This step only takes a few minutes a day, but it may be the most important step toward your success, so follow through with it.

Every time you read your goals, you will experience the same resourceful, productive feelings that you had when you set them. Reading your goals on a daily basis will help you focus for the day ahead, by reminding you of the progress you are making in your approach to eating and exercise. This review will prevent you from slipping back to your old destructive ways. By strengthening your focus, you are able to act more congruently with your wellness intentions, and thus your performance improves. With time, experience, and repetition, you will develop a deep connection to these wellness habits, and they will eventually feel normal to you. The benefits will become more evident and more rewarding as you persevere, and the effort required to remain focused will virtually evaporate.

You will know your wellness habits have become a natural part of your lifestyle if you try going back to your old ways, and they no longer feel natural for you.

Before you move on from goal setting, we want you to specifically outline the personal benefits you will derive from reading your goals everyday and acting congruently to achieve them. By remaining faithful to your workout program, and by satisfying your dietary goals regarding complex carbohydrates, dietary fiber, anti-cancer foods, and low-fat protein foods, what personal benefits are you planning to experience and enjoy? The headings that follow will help you organize your thoughts.

Personal Benefits

External Benefits
If there will be a benefit to your physical appearance, describe what the improvements will be (weight, waistline measurements, etc.):

Internal Benefits
If you are working to lower your risk of certain diseases, what changes will occur within your body to facilitate this outcome? (e.g., lower blood cholesterol = lower heart attack risk)

Intangible Benefits
(these are the ones that you can't measure with a yardstick or blood sample, such as self-esteem, popularity, etc.) Start by answering the following questions.

After filling out the above categories, will you feel better about yourself by taking action to succeed? Yes____ No ____

Do you think that physical wellness will enhance the social dimensions of your life? Yes____ No ____

Is it important to you to live long enough to fully enjoy your children and your grandchildren? Yes____ No ____

What other psychological or intangible benefits will you experience by succeeding with your wellness goals?

Starting Right Now . . .

Read your goals every day. Use them to motivate you into making consistent wellness choices throughout the day.

Summary for Step 4

1. Goal setting is the active step of seeing how the Winning Weigh program will benefit your life.
2. The three parts of goal setting are:
   Part 1 Identify and focus on the areas of your life that you want to change or modify to become more wellness-oriented.
   Part 2 Be specific about what you are going to do to achieve these alterations in your lifestyle.
   Part 3 List the benefits that achieving these goals will bring to your life.
3. Remember: goals only exist if they are written down.
4. Read your goals on a daily basis to recharge your motivation and commitment to long-term success.

Looking Ahead

In Step 4 you set the goals that will allow you to achieve and enjoy your personal benefits. Along the road to wellness that you will follow, you will meet many roadblocks. In Step 5 we will help you identify your own internal obstacles to long-term success. We'll help you adopt a winning attitude that will help you leap over your particular barriers as they appear in your daily life.

STEP 5   JUMPING THE HURDLES

Your Lifestyle Script

Everyone seems to want to be just the right weight, to get their body into better shape, and to have more energy. Everyone wants to avoid heart disease and cancer. You wouldn't have read this far if you didn't want to achieve these goals, so what's holding you back?

You may wonder where you will get the strength to overcome your old desires and habits. You may fear that you won't succeed with the goals you have just set for yourself. Rationally, you may want to be thin, fit, and healthy, but part of you still seems to want to gorge on unhealthy food and lie around. This battle is usually fought in your unconscious mind.

Your Unconscious Mind

Your unconscious mind is a collection of your lifetime experiences, memories, thoughts, and emotions. Miraculously, your unconscious is able to organize all of these pieces of information and experiences into fixed patterns that dictate how you react in different situations. Someone might ask, "Do you like country and western music?" Immediately an answer pops into your mind. You meet someone for the first time and immediately begin to collect opinions and beliefs about the person. Your unconscious mind is constantly evaluating, analyzing, and providing you with a reaction to every single one of life's events. It is your decision-making command center.

Somewhere in your unconscious lies an automated program that defines your relationships with food, exercise, and health. These relationships have developed over your entire lifetime. For example, from the very first moments of your life, feeding, nourishment, and love have been closely tied together. It is not surprising that you turn to food during lonely times, sad times, nervous times, or even happy times. Food has been a lifelong link to your family, community, and friends. That's why you can't alter this relationship overnight with a simple promise to be good forever, starting tomorrow.

Your Lifestyle Script

Have you ever been spellbound by a movie? Even though you rationally know that the actors are following a script, you are right there, caught up in the action. Many good movies pull you into their own spontaneous reality. Watching a movie for a second time, on the other hand, you anticipate your favorite scenes, laugh at punch lines before they are delivered, and no longer shiver at suspenseful parts. Rather than being caught up in the story, your rational mind is available to watch how the movie is put together. You notice the lighting, the music, the special effects. You are able to appreciate the director's role in staging and developing the plot.

Until now, you have been an actor in your own lifestyle script, which may include a weight-loss and weight-gain subplot, a nutrition subplot, and an exercise subplot. Most of the time you spontaneously act out the same scenes, year after year, without any conscious awareness of the script, the plot, or the roles you are playing.

We now want you to get to know your own personal lifestyle script so you can avoid getting caught up in it, so you can become the director instead of one of the characters. Thus, you can overcome the part of your unconscious mind that casts you as being overweight or unhealthy or lazy forever. By recognizing your unconscious role in the script, you can step aside when the old cues are given. Only then will you be able to stop yourself from repeating your unhealthy eating patterns again and again.

One very commom lifestyle script falls into three distinct acts:

Act I: The Blissful Binge
Act II: The Perfect Forever Fantasy
Act III: The Revolution

To explore these acts more closely, we will look at the script in action. Whatever your health goals are – eating more healthy foods, exercising more often, keeping your blood pressure down – the basic plot of the script will be the same. So, as you read the script, ask yourself how it applies to you.

Act I
The Blissful Binge

Scene i
The scene opens on a comfortable living room. You are stretched out on the couch in front of the television. On the coffee table, within easy reach, are potato chips, beer, pop, chocolate cake, and whatever else you could possibly want to eat. Without thinking, you put bite after bite in your mouth as you watch Janet Leigh leave Norman Bates alone with his stuffed birds and step into the shower. The telephone rings at that crucial moment. It is your friend, asking you out for a brisk walk. But no, you have other plans: you have to find out (for the sixth time) who killed poor Janet. After all, maybe this time Norman will go see a psychotherapist and work out his problems with his mother.

Scene ii
Three months later
Same scene as before, same smorgasbord of food, different movie on television. You are still stretched out on the couch, but you are 30 pounds heavier. A commercial for potato chips comes on the television, so you go to the kitchen for more beer. On the way, you pass the full-length mirror hanging in your hall. When you catch sight of your "new" figure (somehow unnoticed for the last three months), disbelief and then panic spread over your face. You run sobbing to the telephone to call your friend, who has just come back from another brisk walk.

You: (still sobbing) I . . . I'm big and fat and . . . and huge. I swear I was all right yesterday. How did I get so fat all of a sudden? What will I do? I'm so ugly. I'll die of a heart attack. Help me!

Friend: (shocked you hadn't noticed earlier that you were putting on weight) Oh . . . well . . . ***you*** know what to do. You have to eat fewer fattening foods and exercise more.

You: (with growing enthusiasm) I will. I will! I'll never, never eat chocolate cake again. I'll never eat anything sweet – who needs it? I'll never even put dressing on my salads! I'll run **ten miles** every day! Let's see . . . I could lose 30 pounds in three weeks. No! I can lose it in **two** weeks. Do you want to run up Mount Upandup with me tomorrow?

Friend: It's pretty steep. I don't think I can run so . . .

You: No! No! I have a better idea. Let's go running the day **after** tomorrow. Tomorrow we'll have a party to celebrate my new lifestyle . . . my new figure. We'll eat all the bad foods we really want to eat **one last time.** We'll get it all out of our systems once and for all! Then we'll go on that diet where you lose three pounds every day by eating nothing but grapefruit.

Friend: (doubtfully) I really don't think that diet is such a good idea.

You: Sure it is! Everything will be fine. See you tomorrow!

Scene iii
The next day
You emerge, relaxed and happy, from a book store with a huge stack of diet and exercise books in your arms. Humming, you enter a pizzeria and order a pizza topped with double cheese, bacon, and fried onions. Next, you go to a pastry shop and come

out with a Danish or two. Balancing your purchases precariously, you buy a bag of chips to eat on the way home. It's a shame your friend didn't want to join you. Suddenly you stop, anxious and worried. You forgot to buy a bottle of pop to wash it all down.

Act II
The Perfect Forever Fantasy

Scene i
The next day
You are sitting eating your breakfast of grapefruit and bean sprouts, feeling a little smug about your tremendous will power and fortitude, when the phone rings. It is your friend, calling to tell you about the fancy dinner she had the night before.

You: What did you eat?

Friend: Lobster, baked potato with a little bit of sour cream, Caesar salad, and sherbet for dessert. It was delicious! Then we danced all evening. I had such a lot of fun.
You: (self-righteously) But those are **bad** foods. Sour cream is full of saturated fats and sherbet is full of sugar. And everyone knows that potatoes are fattening . . . and lobster too! You know better than that.

Friend: (surprised) But you eat worse than I do! You were telling me just last week that we only live once so we might as well eat the foods we like.

You: Not any more! Now I only eat **good** foods. I know I've tried before to change the way I eat, but this time I really mean it. You just have to be self-disciplined. (accusingly) Did you have anything to drink?

Friend: Just a glass of champagne . . .

You: outraged) Champagne!

Scene ii
Three weeks later
You are at the breakfast table again, once more facing a bowl of grapefruit and bean sprouts. You are really getting very tired of grapefruit and you always did hate bean sprouts. Why don't they leave the poor things in peace – let them turn into real beans. The whole thing is beginning to make you feel cranky. Your friend hasn't phoned you this morning (you know you can't really blame her), which makes you feel lonely and abandoned as well as hungry. You are sure no one loves you. They're all just pretending. Then, you remember the cookies you bought just in case your nephew came to visit. Surely *one* cookie wouldn't hurt . . .

Act III
The Revolution

Scene i
The next day
Grapefruit and bean sprouts *again*. You remember how good that cookie was the day before. Maybe you were right . . . after all, you do only live once. People should love you for yourself, not because you're slim and energetic. Defiantly, you throw your grapefruit and bean sprouts in the garbage and get out the ice cream you had tucked away at the back of the freezer for emergencies.

Scene ii
That night
You are stretched out on the couch in front of the television. On the coffee table, within easy reach, are potato chips, beer, pop, chocolate cake, and whatever else you could possibly want to eat. Unthinkingly, you put bite after bite in your mouth as you watch Janet Leigh leave Norman Bates alone with his stuffed birds and step into the shower . . . .

The Never-Ending Cycle

Sure, we exaggerated the script just a little (well, maybe a lot), but you probably recognized parts of it all the same. Our insights into this pattern evolved through our work with patients who had developed serious problems through trying quick-fix diet programs, but most of us show some tendencies to use this pattern.

The diagram in Exhibit 5-1 shows how this lifestyle script is a cycle. You can go round and round that cycle all your life in a frustrating attempt to lose weight, start exercising, or eat more health-promoting foods. In the first part of the cycle, you procrastinate, while eating all the junk food you want and lying around all day. In the second part of the cycle, you deprive yourself of the things you used to indulge in.

Exhibit 5-1
The Blissful Binge/Perfect Forever Cycle

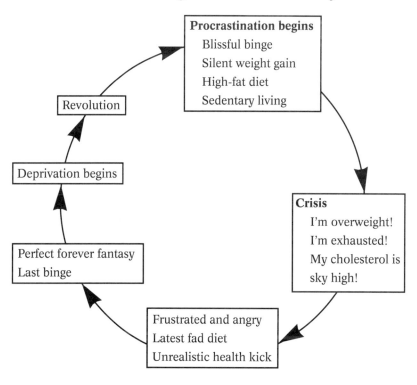

The same common characteristics apply to other wellness challenges. You may have joined a health club at some time in your life. If you were a typical member, you at first committed to several exercise sessions per week, keen to get yourself into shape and get the most from your membership investment. Soon, you missed some sessions because of other commitments or lack of energy, and within a few weeks you were a member in name only. Your resolve may have been renewed when you got tired after climbing a couple of flights of stairs or found that the slacks you wore last summer had become too tight. Your renewed enthusiasm may have been so strong that you injured yourself by trying too hard or you may have grown frustrated that you couldn't keep up the pace you had set for yourself. You stopped exercising again. This sedentary slide followed by a burst of perfect-forever enthusiasm sets up a pattern of procrastination followed by unrealistic enthusiasm. Without some realistic goals and some psychological preparation, this cycle could go on forever.

You may have found out at some point that you have a high blood cholesterol level. You immediately may have tried to cut your fat intake from 35 percent to 5 percent. Inevitably, you began to resent the restrictions. Sometimes you slipped entirely and had 50 percent fat days. Over the long term, you may have found that you ended up eating almost as much fat as you used to eat. We will try to help you establish a more reasonable pattern for fat reduction that will let you enjoy the new you rather than fighting to resist your temptations.

Surprisingly, in the blissful binge stage or your personal equivalent, you don't usually recognize that you have let your health slide until some critical moment. You may notice those extra pounds when passing by a full-length mirror or when trying on old clothes. You may run for a bus one day, only to find yourself sweating and exhausted after only half a block. Maybe your doctor tells you your cholesterol is too high or that your blood pressure has shot through the roof. Eventually ***something*** wakes you from your blissful binge. Then you panic and decide you need to do something about it overnight.

The typical reaction to a newly discovered bulging figure is the immediate elimination of all the high fat or simple sugar foods you have been enjoying for months. You adopt the latest "last chance" diet, on which you are "guaranteed" to lose a lot of weight very quickly. If you are out of shape, you start training for the marathon the next day. Thus, you go from a binge approach to a perfect forever approach in less than 24 hours. Obviously, if you are starting a lifetime of deprivation, you deserve one last pig-out. Blissfully, you sleep through the night awakening to the start of Act II.

During Act II, the perfect forever fantasy, you are sure you won't give in to your destructive eating habits or abandon your exercise habits. You take pride in your will power, fortitude, and self-control. You preach the values of weight loss and the evils of the North American diet to everyone you meet. You speak of the "bad foods" that clog your arteries and produce cancer. You exercise every day, making sure to let *everyone* know how hard you are working. You may recognize that you've played this role before and failed. Sadly, you are so self-righteous in your perfect forever fantasy scene that you honestly believe you really mean it this time.

Notice that during Act II, you label foods and behavior as being "good" or "bad." You pledge to be good forever and always to stay away from bad food. ***Ironically, it is the very act of swearing off bad activities that results in your eventual failure.*** Swearing off bad foods and suppressing your desire for them takes a great deal of unconscious energy. The more you push away your old desires for bad foods, the more frustrated, irritable, and deprived you feel. The more you stress will power and fortitude, the more desirable the foods you are denying yourself will seem. Eventually, you might have a cookie or a small piece of cake. Or, you might have a cold and not be able to exercise for a while. Overnight you enter the third act . . . the revolution.

A revolution in your mind is not much different from a revolution in a country: one group has been suppressing another group's freedom to do as it likes and the other group gets fed up. You have imposed a famine on yourself, censoring any desires for "bad foods" or for lying around taking it easy. Your unconscious mind feels suppressed because it can't think or eat or behave as it likes, and a battle develops between the feast and famine parts of you. Thoughts like "I only live once, so why don't I just enjoy myself?" give warning of the impending revolution. Eventually, it only takes one small snack to give your blissful binge revolutionaries enough strength to overthrow your perfect forever dictator.

Then, welcome back to Act I — the blissful binge.

No Damage Done? Wrong!

Besides the physiological problems of continually losing and regaining weight, starting and stopping an exercise program, or treating high blood pressure intermittently, there is also a significant psychological impact from the kind of lifestyle script we have just described. The three-act lifestyle script becomes more and more automatic. Eventually, it takes less of a struggle to switch from Act I to Act II to Act III, and soon the story line develops a life of its own. Unconsciously, you begin to base all your health choices on either a perfect forever or blissful binge approach. So, you either end up feeling fat, lazy, and apathetic or frustrated, self-righteous, and deprived. These two approaches are shown graphically in Exhibit 5-2.

Exhibit 5–2
Two Approaches to Health

The Blissful Binge Approach

- blissful
- eating "bad" foods
- sedentary
- feeling apathetic
- feeling free to do as you like the "right" thing
- out of control
- overweight and unhealthy
- scornful of anyone who watches out for his or her health
- a Sedentary Slob

The Perfect Forever Approach

- fanatical
- eating "good" foods
- driven to exercise
- feeling deprived
- feeling obligated to do
- overcontrolled
- repressed and miserable
- resentful of anyone who enjoys a treat or a day off
- a Self-Righteous Snob

Your Role in Your Lifestyle Script

By exploring your own unique lifestyle script, you will be able to break out of your unconscious, automatic pattern of alternating between the perfect forever approach and the blissful binge approach. In each of these approaches, you play a different character, or role.

The concept of a role is a simple one. Looking at your own life, you will realize that you act, feel, and think differently when you are in different situations. You play different roles as a sibling, a parent, a son or daughter, a lover, a boss, and an employee. You are not a different person, but there is a subtle shift of emphasis in the part of your personality that you show. A role is a collection of thoughts, feelings, beliefs, and memories that are activated by a given experience or situation.

Who Was That Last Night Anyway?

How often have you asked yourself that question? Have you ever seemed to be possessed late at night by an impulsive side of yourself that took over and guided your behavior? Mysteriously, your memory of an eating binge may be hazy or clouded. You certainly know that you ate the food, but you may have felt little pleasure or enjoyment. For most people, it is a hurried, tense indulgence.

The reason that your memory is fuzzy and lacks detail by the next morning is that during the night you made a transition from one role to another. It is not surprising that you feel disconnected from the experience of the night before.

In your personal lifestyle script, you act out different roles in each of the different acts. During a binge, in Act I, you are playing the helpless, impulsive role we call the Sedentary Slob. By the next morning, you may have returned to playing the obedient Self-Righteous Snob from Act II. It is not surprising that, speaking as the Self-Righteous Snob, you'd ask the question, "Who was that last night anyway?" Your impulsive Sedentary Slob role is already tucked away in your unconscious mind.

Most of the patients we see in our practices follow some version of a lifestyle script with their own personalized versions of the Sedentary Slob and the Self-Righteous Snob. KP, a 37-year-old commercial artist, is a typical example. She had been flipping back and forth between the Sedentary Slob and Self-Righteous Snob roles for years. For months at a time, she would eat only the right foods. One percent yogurt was too high in fat for her; eating a cookie was unthinkable. She rode ten miles on her exercise bicycle every day without fail and preached fanatically to everyone about the evils of their diets. This perfectionist pattern would last about four months – until she had lost 30 pounds and brought her blood pressure down. Then, inevitably, she would begin to resent her restrictive lifestyle.

Eventually, something would go wrong. Once she got the flu and couldn't exercise for a week. Another time, she broke down and had a piece of cake on her birthday. Some little incident would get her off track and she'd slip back into her Sedentary Slob role. She couldn't even bring herself to *sit* on her exercise bicycle. The staff at the convenience store got to know her by name because she'd come in daily to stock up on junk food. She felt as if she couldn't do anything right, she was losing her self-confidence at work, and she didn't believe she would ever get into shape again. Quickly, she would regain all the weight she had lost and then some.

During her therapy, we focused on finding a balance point between these two extremes. She came to recognize her two roles and to understand that both of them were unhealthy. She named them the "Helpless Wimp" and the "Wicked Witch." We encouraged her to take a more self-supportive, less punishing approach, and she was gradually able to be comfortable with a more moderate and flexible health program. Now, she does not swear off a long list foods forever and she exercises for 30 minutes only four times a week. She has found her own equilibrium point, based on her personal wellness goals, and she manages to be healthy *and* happy – both at the same time.

You can see that neither her Helpless Wimp nor her

Wicked Witch role gave KP much chance for long-term success. The overly restrictive lifestyle dictated by the Self-Righteous Snob merely forced the Sedentary Slob to demand equal time. Eventually, it would explode back to the surface with even more force than before. In order to stop the lifetime up-and-down approach to wellness and weight loss, you have to step back, recognize the role you are playing, and find the middle ground where *you* feel comfortable.

Your Sedentary Slob

Your Sedentary Slob role contributes most to your failure to attain your wellness goals. Your Sedentary Slob has thoughts like

"I'll never succeed, so why bother trying?"
or
"I need a doughnut to cheer me up."
or
"I shouldn't exercise today. What I really need after a long day behind a desk is to lie down for awhile."

Your Sedentary Slob role is most active late at night, in stressful situations, and when you're feeling bored. One of our patients described how she experiences her Sedentary Slob:

> This is the part of me that feels so fat. It's the part of me that's present late at night after my boss yells at me or when I'm tired in the late afternoon. In this role, I gobble food, eating alone, stuffing down two chocolate bars without seeing if I like the taste. After an entire evening of doing well at a party, I will automatically switch into this role at the end of the night and begin to move from table to table, sampling and taste-testing all the leftover goodies. You'd think I was a human vacuum cleaner!

> To begin to break out of your lifestyle script, you have to learn to recognize your Sedentary Slob. Then, you will be ready for it when it becomes active.

Starting Right Now . . .

Watch for your own version of the lifestyle script. Focus on spotting signs of your own Sedentary Slob or your Self-Righteous Snob roles. Whenever you see yourself slipping into one of these automatic unconscious roles, follow these steps:

1. Recognize where you are in your script.
2. Take a slow, deep breath, filling your lungs.
3. Smile at how you have slipped into a familiar role and roll your shoulders back slowly.
4. Take another deep breath.
5. Decide what you would like to do, taking into account your personal goals.
6. Whatever you choose, be content with your decision.

By following this process, you begin to short-circuit your automatic reactions. If you step back from the script and smile at how it is unfolding, you will no longer be completely caught up in your role.

Answer the questions in the Wellness Planner (pages 315-316) to get a better idea of your own lifestyle script and Sedentary Slob.

Recognizing Your Sedentary Slob

Your Sedentary Slob can be found at places all along your wellness journey. The long-distance runner who is tempted to stop before reaching the finish line is hearing the voice of his or her Sedentary Slob. So are early morning exercisers who promise themselves they will work out later in the day. If you ignore that voice and keep running or get out of bed anyway, you will often find that the run and the day provide extra satisfaction. This chapter will help you overcome your Sedentary Slob, even while you accept its presence.

You have begun to recognize your lifestyle script and to see the roles that your Sedentary Slob and Self-Righteous Snob play. The Sedentary Slob and Self-Righteous Snob are parts of the whole you, but you are capable of stepping back and watching yourself act out those parts. To avoid getting trapped in these roles, you must learn to recognize what situations bring them to the surface and what you believe and how you think at these moments.

We will talk mostly about your Sedentary Slob, since that is the most destructive role. Usually your Self-Righteous Snob disappears naturally as you begin to follow your wellness goals. Since Winning Weigh wellness goals are based on your personal version of the program, the perfect forever fantasy act of your lifestyle script is easily replaced by a balanced wellness approach. However, you should remember that your Self-Righteous Snob undermines your wellness goals just as completely as your Sedentary Slob does. Swearing off "bad" behavior for the rest of your life inevitably leads to yearning for the banned foods and eventual rebelling against your goals. The way to wellness is not to switch from your Sedentary Slob to your Self-Righteous Snob, but to find a place in the middle from which you can make conscious decisions about your health.

Sedentary Slob Activators

Certain situations automatically summon up your Sedentary Slob. Once it has taken over the stage, you have certain thoughts and feelings and, inevitably, you carry out certain repetitive actions. You may eat a frozen dessert or gulp down a container of ice cream while watching a late-night movie. You may decide you are too tired to exercise. By discovering the triggers that activate your Sedentary Slob, you can develop an early warning system that will give you time to disconnect yourself from the role so that you don't automatically carry out destructive behavior.

An activator is a cue that awakens a specific role. Your Sedentary Slob is lying dormant in your unconscious, waiting for an appropriate trigger so it can rise up and run your life. A common trigger for adults is visiting their parents' home. As soon as they walk into the house, they automatically open the refrigerator door and snack on a few choice items. Many people don't even realize they've done it. Returning to their childhood home is an activator that reawakens an earlier pattern of eating behavior.

Look on these activators as red flags, warning you that a crisis is coming. Once you know these situations are coming, you can develop strategies for dealing with them.

There are three main categories of activators: situations, people, and energy states. As you read about each of these categories, think about what your own triggers might be.

Activator Category No. 1: Situations

A situation activator is a specific circumstance or combination of events that triggers your Sedentary Slob. Some examples given by our patients are

- getting up on a winter morning and getting on the stationary bicycle
- sitting alone at night
- watching a favorite TV show
- watching commercials for junk food
- coming home late from work to an empty house
- making dinner for the family
- finishing a hard day at work
- paying bills or doing laundry
- going out with friends
- enjoying a wedding, bar mitzvah, party, or even the weekend
- working out after a long workday

Activator Category No. 2: People

Some people make you feel the need to be fed or babied. Probably a whole series of people in your life can activate your Sedentary Slob by their presence, absence, or comments. Here are some examples from our clients:

- jogging with a friend who runs a mile a minute faster than me
- my boss, when he yells at me
- my mother, who makes me angry
- my friend, who says I am no fun since I went on this fanatical health kick
- my bridge group, when it is cancelled
- my family, when I visit for the holidays
- my ex, when I have to talk to him or her
- my girlfriend, when I don't see her for a couple of days

Activator Cateory No. 3: Energy States

Your energy state is your general feeling of well-being. A low energy state puts you at risk of easily slipping into your Sedentary Slob role. The following list shows some of the feelings that can bring on the Sedentary Slob:

- fatigue or tiredness
- anxiety
- sadness or nervousness
- boredom
- wanting to avoid an unpleasant task
- loneliness and feeling unloved

Many of these feelings are such common triggers for food that we often forget that food isn't really what we want. When we are lonely, we eat instead of calling a friend. When we are tired, we eat instead of taking a nap. An anxious, low-energy state is an especially powerful activator because food will actually calm you. However, it is only one of many ways of changing your mood. By recognizing your energy states, you can develop non-food solutions to these everyday obstacles.

For example, use exercise or a power nap to switch out of your tired energy state. Take careful note of your thoughts before and after you exercise and you will see how aerobic exercise literally changes your mood, rescuing you from your Sedentary Slob.

Once you recognize what your activators are, you can begin to identify what they activate – your Sedentary Slob. If you see yourself as helpless when you are in your Sedentary Slob role, then you act helpless. The role is often so engrained that you are unable to step back and question whether or not they are valid, legitimate, or even real!

The first step to greater freedom is to step back and get to know this automatic, unconscious mentality. Explore your personal lifestyle script. Imagine your Sedentary Slob as someone you are meeting for the first time. Get to know what it feels, thinks, and believes about life. Its specific feelings, thoughts, and beliefs guide *your* wellness habits.

Your Sedentary Slob Beliefs

We all live with a multitude of beliefs that we use to organize the world. Discovering your beliefs is difficult. You can try asking open-ended questions about how you feel about specific subjects. Whatever thoughts automatically come to mind are your beliefs.

Without discovering your unique beliefs, you'll never be able to give up the rules you live by. One patient explained to me why she liked chocolate cake. She said, "My grandmother used to serve me cake in her apartment. She'd sit there with a warm smile and loving eyes while I drank my milk and ate the cake." Until she'd explored what she really believed about cake, she hadn't realized what it meant to her: it was the bridge to an important, loving figure in her life. Because she now consciously realized what cake meant to her, the next time she felt lonely and unloved, she could change the scripts. Instead of reaching for cake, she thought warmly of her grandmother.

Let's look at some of the common ways people complete open-ended sentences about their wellness beliefs. "Fat people are..." usually gets responses like "lazy, weak, unmotivated, out of control, satisfied, lonely, depressed, jolly, ugly, stupid, good in bed, and fat forever." Your responses give you a glimpse of how you see yourself and how you behave as the Sedentary Slob. For example, if you believe fat people are unmotivated or ugly, you can't help living this when you are in your Sedentary Slob role.

Typical completions to "Dieting is . . ." include "gross, disgusting, restrictive, a waste of time, stupid, punishing, and always unsuccessful." These are typical beliefs that our patients have when they begin diet programs. These beliefs about dieting translate into irritation and frustration about being on a diet. It's no wonder most diets fail!

According to our patients, healthy foods are good, boring, green, tasteless, horrible, unsatisfying, not filling, and dumb. Beliefs about "good" foods are an important part of your Self-Righteous Snob mode. Because you associate healthy foods with restrictive dieting, you see them negatively. Yet these beliefs aren't true!

In contrast, unhealthy foods are bad, exciting, fun, happy, tasty, satisfying, sweet, greasy, and chocolatey. Chances are that "bad" foods are one of your pleasures. They are treasured in your unconscious, yet in your lifestyle script, you banished them forever. No wonder you are sad and feel like you've lost an old friend! How else would you feel about losing something you call "fun, happy, and exciting"?

Stand back for a moment and realize that unhealthy foods are not necessarily fun, just as healthy foods are not necessarily boring. If you continue to be affected by these beliefs, it will be difficult to feel satisfied while eating a boring "good" food.

Your Thoughts: A Product of Beliefs

Your thoughts are a product of your unconscious beliefs. Let's use a late night snack as an example of the connection between your beliefs and your automatic thoughts.

> It's late at night, and you've been watching a rerun for the fourth time. You're bored and you want to do something fun. It so happens that you've just made a pledge to your latest famine program – the Last Hope Diet.

Suddenly, a random thought pops into your mind: "Have something to eat . . . defrost a frozen cake." You never actually defrost it because you eat it frozen.

In this situation, you need to recognize the automatic thoughts that took place before the idea of a frozen cake popped into your head. This series of thoughts might have gone like this:

1. I'm bored.
2. I'm restless.

These two thoughts activate the unconscious belief that "bad" foods would spice up the evening. This belief results in a third thought:

3. I'll have a treat – there's a cake in the freezer.

Being aware of your thought patterns gives you another opportunity for getting to know your Sedentary Slob. Your challenge is to begin to recognize, become aware of, and even laugh at how your automatic thoughts affect your actions and behavior. Once you do this, you can begin to break free of your automatic behavior, because *you can't both reflect on a role and play the role in the same moment.* You can't be completely involved in behaving like a Sedentary Slob if you are focusing on discovering and exploring your Sedentary Slob's thoughts and beliefs. As soon as you begin to analyze, you are weakening your Sedentary Slob's hold on you. This small separation of yourself from the role provides you with a window of opportunity for long-term change.

Let's take a look at one of the most common automatic thoughts: "I'll eat what I want tonight, but starting tomorrow. . . " You can see the feast followed by the famine built right into that statement. It plays right into your lifestyle scripts. For years you've made this promise to yourself and never kept it. *You cannot make this type of promise and succeed at wellness.* So when you recognize this pattern, seize the moment by recognizing your Sedentary Slob. Then act differently.

Here are ten of the most common thinking styles that reinforce and perpetuate the Sedentary Slob or Self-Righteous Snob roles. As you read about these styles, try to identify how they apply to your lifestyle script.

1. Procrastinated Success

The Procrastinated Success thinking style allows you to delay starting your wellness program. The character Wimpy from the comic strip "Popeye" uses this thinking style. He says, "I'll gladly pay you on Tuesday for a hamburger today." In your lifestyle script, you too take what you want now in exchange for a distant sacrifice that somehow you never get around to making. By the next morning, the taste of the cake is long gone. Immediately, you resent your promise, and rationalize why you can't keep it. Here are some examples of Procrastinated Success thinking:

> I'll start tomorrow.
> I might as well enjoy the wedding first and begin in the morning.
> I'll eat a big dinner tonight and then fast all day tomorrow.
> I'll just eat whatever I want until midnight, and then . . .
> It's September 15th; I'll start a new program on the first of October.
> I'll sleep in instead of going to the gym, but I'll exercise after dinner.

2. Feeling Forecasting

You're using Feeling Forecasting thinking when you get that frightening gut feeling that your present situation will just continue and get worse. In this state, you are so caught up in your feelings of anxiety, frustration, or hopelessness that you belive that they will last forever. Typical Feeling Forecasting thoughts include

> I know even if I lower my fat intake, my cholesterol won't come down.
> I can tell if I get on the bike, I can't do a half hour.
> If I don't eat, I'll just get more and more anxious.
> I know I'm going to end up eating anyway, so this is all a waste.

It is not surprising that, when you think like this, you end up feeling even *more* anxious. Actually, these feelings, along with the crisis that caused them, usually pass quickly. It is only when you struggle with them, using the Feeling Forecasting thinking style, that you intensify and magnify these feelings.

Let's take a closer look at a common Feeling Forecasting statement: "If I don't eat the cookies, I'll just get more and more nervous. In the end, I'll be completely out of control." Notice that there are two basic parts to this thinking style:

- You feel **helpless** and unable to do anything about your situation.
- You feel **hopeless**, believing that the crisis will continue forever unless you give in to the pressure. Inevitably, you do something to relieve the anxiety.

3. Disaster Thinking

The Disaster thinking style is most active after you've had a high-fat snack, munched a doughnut on the run, or missed your exercise session. Suddenly you see yourself as a complete failure – unable to achieve the health goals you set for yourself. Instead of viewing your indulgence as a minor setback, you see yourself condemned to a life of slovenly ill-health. The graph in Exhibit 5–3 illustrates how one patient, who had been successfully following the Winning Weigh program until this point, saw herself after eating five cookies. One five-cookie snack was equal, in her mind, to three weeks of dedication. This is the Disaster thinking style, which punishes you severely for a minor disease-promoting choice.

Exhibit 5-3
Psychological Experience of Success

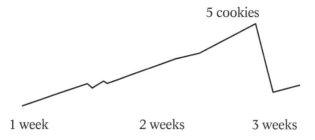

Some common Disaster thoughts are

> I'm so hopeless... I can't even stay on a program for three weeks.
> I'm so pathetic... What kind of eater am I?
> I'm completely out of control.

All of these thoughts can make you give up on your wellness program altogether. However, your Daily Food, Fiber, and Activity Journal can be a real asset in fighting against this kind of thinking style. It allows you to be objective about your progress. By checking your records, you'll see the five cookies for what they really are: a minor setback in a lifetime approach to living.

4. Blaming Others

Blaming Others is such an ingrained and common thinking style, especially when it comes to eating habits, that most of us don't realize when we apply it. The excuses for slipping from a wellness program include business meetings, restaurants with poor menus, weddings, health clubs that are closed on Sundays, Fridays, and rain. Such excuses are all attempts to focus the blame or problem on a source outside yourself. If you tend to use such excuses, remember that at some point you *chose* to do what you did.

5. Blaming Yourself

The Blaming Yourself thinking style appears, on the surface, to be a "helpful" confession of your evil ways. Ironically, it is really a sneaky way to give yourself permission to cheat! Before eating a mound of chocolate ice cream or missing your aerobics class, don't you often blame and chastise yourself for being hopeless, helpless, and weak? By labelling yourself like this, you give yourself permission to cheat on your wellness program. What else could a weak, helpless, and hopeless person do but give in to destructive desires and urges?

6. Weak and Dizzy

Weak and Dizzy can be the most damaging thinking style, keeping you hostage to your old ways. When your Sedentary Slob is most active, you will find yourself too weak and dizzy to follow your wellness program.

While sitting comfortably and reading this book, it is easy to nod in agreement with everything we are saying. Sadly, in the crisis moment, it's easier to think, "I'm just too tired to follow this Winning Weigh program." Other thoughts typical of your Weak and Dizzy thinking style include

> I know this program won't work for me. I'm just too far gone.
> How can I even think in my condition? I am beyond help.

If you use this thinking style, you probably have a dozen more of these excuses on the tip of your tongue.

The Weak and Dizzy thinking style affects your success most strongly because you feel unable to remember the techniques you need to succeed. Weak and Dizzy can also be used in conjunction with any of the other thinking styles. Even after recognizing and labelling your current thinking style, your Weak and Dizzy approach will have you convinced that you are unable to do anything about it.

7. Never, Ever Again

How often have you said, "Starting now, I'll never, ever, do that again"? Very soon, however, you have reverted to the same old pattern.

The very moment you say "never, ever again," you begin a pattern of thinking that increases the value of the banned behavior in your unconscious mind. Swearing off the offending behavior seems to be an appropriate punishment for falling off the wagon. But the cliché "absence makes the heart grow fonder" doesn't just apply to lovers; it also applies to some of your most reliable friends – your bad habits.

PG, a 34-year-old lawyer, used to eat a Mars bar every day. He loved sitting in his office, unwrapping it, and savoring it. His family doctor told him he needed to lose ten pounds. On a Sunday, as a last good-bye, he had two Mars bars. Starting Monday, he cut out chocolate ... for ever and ever. By Friday, he was so anxious that he rushed down to the store and devoured two bars.

Each time you hear yourself saying "never, ever again," you can be sure of one thing – the food or activity you banish will be back; the wellness program you promise to follow forever will be abandoned. In fact, on any new program, if you plan to do too much at the beginning, you have a better chance of failing.

8. And They Lived Happily Ever After
After being in any perfect forever fantasy for a week or so, you'll find yourself having thoughts like

> Well, I'm finally on the right track forever.
> Finally, I have the will power to succeed.

With thoughts like these, it is not surprising that you are devastated when you finally indulge in a "banned" food or activity. By being harsh with yourself, you sabotage your program and go back to your old ways.

9. Doing/Undoing
The Doing/Undoing thinking style applies to you if you live out lifestyle scripts on a daily basis. Do you have a cigarette on the way to the health club or eat ice cream after refusing salad dressing at lunch? This contradictory behavior – doing the wellness thing and then undoing it again – leads to a yoyo effect. Instead of following a middle-of-the-road

approach, you alternate between being "very, very good" and "very, very bad." This back-and-forth pattern will continue until you recognize it and set realistic goals.

10. Eureka

You slip into the Eureka thinking style every time you react to a book, product, idea, ad, or fact by saying, "Finally, I've found the answer." Perhaps an ad promises, "Recently discovered herb allows you to get aerobic exercise from the comfort of your living room chair" or "Lose ten pounds a week and never be hungry again." Later, in the fine print, you find out that it only works if you slip into a coma first. If you hear something that sounds too good to be true and you feel that thrill of excitement, think again. You'll lose in the long run by putting your faith in schemes that are bound to fail.

Exhibit 5–4
Ten Thinking Styles

1. Procrastinated Success
2. Feeling Forecasting
3. The Fat Boy/Fat Girl
4. Blaming Others
5. Blaming Yourself
6. Weak and Dizzy
7. Never, Ever Again
8. And They Lived Happily Ever After
9. Doing/Undoing
10. Eureka

Changing Your Thinking Style

If you find yourself using one of your Sedentary Slob's thinking styles, then follow these three steps:

1. Identify what situations, people, or feelings activated the thought.

2. Listen to the thought. You can even take notes if it helps. For many people, the writing helps them step out of their thinking style.

3. Label the thinking style. Remember that simply observing automatic behavior consciously helps you to break free of it. You can't both study a role and play it at the same time. So decide which of the ten thinking styles applies to your own personal thoughts. If none do, then make up your own.

Starting Right Now . . .

1. Make a list of your Sedentary Slob activators in your Wellness Planner (p. 317). Take note of the people in your life who can set off your Sedentary Slob. Focus on what they say or do that motivates your desire for destructive behavior.

2. Continue to look out for activators and add them to your list. Each day presents opportunities for recognizing new activators. You should also become more sensitive to the details of the activators you have already identified. You might discover that your Sedentary Slob is not activated by your friend Jill herself, but by her weekly advice that you'd be happier if you were in a committed relationship. This type of specific detail gives you greater ability to disconnect your Sedentary Slob before it begins to dictate your behavior.

3. Take note of any new situations, people, energy states, or thoughts that increase your desire to subvert your wellness goals. Remember to be as detailed and specific as possible when you record your activators.

4. Use the Wellness Planner (p. 318) to explore your beliefs about wellness by using open-ended questions. The better you understand the beliefs of your Sedentary Slob and Self-Righteous Snob, the better you can avoid automatic, destructive behavior.

5. In the Wellness Planner (p. 319), collect samples of your automatic thoughts and identify which thinking style applies to each one. The better you understand the way you think, the more easily you can change it.

Adopting a Winning Attitude

Now that you are acquainted with your lifestyle script and your Sedentary Slob, you can begin to adopt a winning attitude. Your attitude is the way you see the world – whether you consider the glass to be half full or half empty. A winning attitude is the belief that you can and will succeed at your goals. A positive attitude will fuel your commitment and encourage you to make health-promoting choices.

You may believe that people either grow up with a positive attitude or they don't. You may believe that having a winning attitude depends on the circumstances of your life or on your luck. In fact, for most people, a winning attitude doesn't come without effort. Usually, you have to *adopt* a winning attitude consciously. It's a little like adopting a child. With time, love, belief in yourself as a parent, and hard work, the child becomes yours – your own flesh and blood. Notice those four important ingredients: love, time, belief in yourself, and hard work.

Love

To get in touch with the wellness part of yourself and to adopt a new attitude, you must first love the you that you are right now. On the wellness ladder, you may find yourself criticizing yourself often, hoping to see Jane Fonda in the mirror instead of yourself. No loving mother would tell her child, "Bob's a good boy – not like you. I wish he were my son." You have to learn to be as accepting of yourself.

Have compassion for the person you are at this very moment. Would you demand that a toddler read? Life is an ongoing process of growth. Feel love for yourself at the stage you are in *now.* This compassion and love is important if you are to succeed at developing a winning attitude.

Time

There are many types of time. The type closely connected to your Sedentary Slob is procrastinated, endless time. This time has no beginning and no end. You plan to begin each task tommorrow, never today. The journey will begin at any moment except *this* moment.

The Self-Righteous Snob has its own type of time. Here there is a definite beginning but also an abrupt end. This time is based on reaching a destination, but ends suddenly with a binge or minor setback.

Winning-attitude time has a long-range perspective. It is divided into small units but is open-ended in duration. It's an endless journey with specific stops along the way. Each of these specific stops represents a destination, a target for accomplishment. By setting goals at the end of each unit of time, but knowing that each goal is simply the beginning of the next goal, you can avoid that unreachable-destination feeling of the Self-Righteous Snob that signals the beginning of the end; yet, unlike the Sedentary Snob, you can get started and get motivated.

Belief in Yourself

By setting realistic goals and then believing that you can accomplish them, you are on your way to success. This belief in yourself is crucial to developing a winning attitude. It means that you expect to achieve wellness. To believe in yourself means first loving yourself as you are in this moment, then creating a realistic plan, and finally dedicating yourself to nurturing a new you.

Hard Work

Wherever you look in life, you'll see that you cannot accomplish anything in the long run without effort and sacrifice, so why should you think that good health will not require an investment? Many people are willing to work very hard almost every day of their lives to achieve a particular level of income and financial security. Building relationships with people you love also requires effort and hard work. The same is true for preserving your health. If wellness seems worthwhile to you, then the price of achieving health goals should seem small by comparison with the value you purchase through that effort. Only you can truly decide on the importance of health in your life. That is why any goal you set must be your goal – a reflection of your philosophy, attitudes, and long-term plans. We can tell you from first-hand experience that if you begin now to follow the Winning Weigh program, you are almost certain to discover that you will become happier as your health and appearance improve. With time, the price will seem smaller and the sacrifices less significant. The benefits, on the other hand, will seem more and more worthwhile.

Breathing and Posturizing: The Mind-Body Link

The ways you breathe and carry yourself influence your attitude. In the chapter on lifestyle scripts, we explored the thoughts, feelings, and unconscious story line of the Sedentary Slob. You need to disconnect yourself from that role. You probably recognize that when you feel anxious, depressed, or angry, you are more likely to eat disease-promoting foods or skip your exercise workout. You may not realize that there is a connection between your breathing, gestures, and posture and the anxiety, depression, and anger you sometimes feel. Usually your mood determines these characteristics, but you can learn to use the connection the other way.

Actors use their breathing, gestures, and posture to convey to the audience how they are feeling. You also use postures, facial expressions, and breathing patterns, often unconsciously, that demonstrate ***and help create*** how you are feeling.

Let's look at an example. One of our patients, MJ, was a 54-year-old woman who gorged herself nightly after her family went to bed. She'd be reading in the living room when she'd feel herself drawn to the kitchen. The closer she got, the more anxious she'd ***feel.*** Once she started exploring her body language, she noticed that in this state her shoulders rounded, her body slouched over, and her breathing became shallow and rapid. Her body was saying she was frightened of her urge to eat. Once in the kitchen, she would quickly shove the food into her mouth, hunched over the plate in a daze.

MJ's posture and breathing were important parts of her Sedentary Slob role. By modifying her posture and breathing, she was able to step out of that role and make a conscious decision. To break the hold of her Sedentary Slob, she used two important techniques: diaphragmatic breathing and posturizing.

Diaphragmatic Breathing

Most people believe that they are fairly competent at breathing. After all, they have been doing it all their lives. They don't know, however, that by changing the way they breathe, they can change the way they feel and think. In fact, control of breathing is the basis of many meditation and modern relaxation techniques.

In this section, we will describe a special type of breathing, called ***diaphragmatic breathing.*** Your diaphragm is an important part of your breathing apparatus. You use it for the deep, final portion of each breath. During even mildly anxious moments, you stop using your diaphragm. You breathe more shallowly, without using the deep recesses of your chest. Filling your entire chest is the key to breaking the patterns that promote stress. Here is the basic technique:

1. Sit as comfortably as possible and close your eyes. Place your right hand on your chest and your left hand on your abdomen at your navel.

2. Take deep breaths that make your left (lower) hand rise much more than your right (chest) hand rises.

3. As you continue to take slow, deep breaths, repeat these words slowly and rhythmically in time with your breathing: "Cool air in (as you breath in). Warm air out (as you breath out)." This will help regulate the speed with which you breathe.

Initially, you may feel a tightness in your throat or a nervous feeling in your chest or back when you take a deep breath. This feeling will disappear as you practice diaphragmatic breathing.

You may feel that you cannot breathe in more deeply, even before your chest is expanded. Gently push on with your effort and breathe as much air as you can so you will gain the full benefits of diaphragmatic breathing.

To really master this important technique, you'll need to practice for a few minutes each day. If you don't close your eyes, you can practice anywhere. One psychologist friend of ours likes to say,

"When I'm driving, a red light means 'go' for diaphragmatic breathing." Each time she comes to a red light, she uses the time to practice her breathing. Do it in your office, at meetings, in bed, or anywhere else that an uncomfortable feeling hits you. Once you master the technique, even two or three deep breaths can clear away anxiety. Some professionals who teach breathing techniques use a single deep breath as an "on" switch for relaxation.

Posturizing

Posturizing helps you to break out of the physical posture and facial expression of your Sedentary Slob. By altering your body position and movements in a positive way, you can change your body's physiology and internal chemistry. This physical change in turn helps to create a positive state of mind and positive behavior changes. Use the posturizing technique whenever you feel yourself slipping into a disease-promoting choice. It's especially important when you need time out – a breathing space in which to make a conscious wellness decision rather than automatically acting out an old script. Posturizing is part of the mind-body connection. It will help you escape an "I'm going to fail" attitude and replace it with a winning attitude and a healthier approach to living. Follow these three simple steps:

1. As you take a deep breath, gently roll your shoulders back.

2. Take a second deep breath, lifting your head, rolling back your shoulders again, and stretching your body up towards the sky without lifting your arms.

3. End with another deep breath and a smile.

Visualizing a New You

After a lifetime of Sedentary Slob excuses and failures, it is time to renew your lost love affair with your body. Visualization is one of the critical ingredients for reawakening and developing your wellness attitudes and beliefs. Instead of just reading over your goals, plans, and solutions, you create, in your imagination, a detailed image of your success. Visualizing is the natural complement to setting goals. Goal setting strengthens your thinking mind while visualizing encourages your emotions and enthusiasm. Your feelings are not only the basis of your lifestyle script; they are also the source of your will to succeed.

Visualization is like active daydreaming – you create the story line, determine the outcome, and imagine the personal benefits. By actively seeing yourself succeeding at your goals and overcoming any obstacles in your mind's eye, you create a unconscious library of successful wellness choices. These images will fuel your desire, courage, and enthusiasm to free yourself from the clutches of your Sedentary Slob and Self-Righteous Snob. You will inevitably find it easier in high-anxiety moments to make health-promoting choices.

After practicing visualization for a few weeks, you will begin to experience a deeper sense of commitment to your day-to-day wellness choices. More of your unconscious energy will be directed towards your conscious goals. You will develop the mental muscles you need to overcome your automatic Sedentary Slob impulses.

Relaxation

Visualization is performed in a relaxed, meditative state. In fact, being relaxed is critical to visualizing effectively. Relaxation is simply an energy state, one possible level of emotional vigor. Your energy state, or the way you feel about an event, has a profound effect on your attitude, on whether you see the glass as half empty or half full. Because you are relaxed when you visualize a situation, you invest it with this serene feeling. When you are faced with the actual situation, you are more likely to be calm and relaxed then as well. Your visualization period is a dress rehearsal. Relaxation is important because the neural pathways that are laid down are more effective when you are relaxed.

When first trying a relaxation technique, many people become anxious and struggle with thoughts like, "Am I doing this right?" That's OK Accept your tension. Simply acknowledge your inner concern, take a deep breath, and return to the relaxation exercise. It is your ability to return to the exercise, despite your noisy inner voices, that allows you to relax. No one does these exercises perfectly.

Our relaxation technique is really just an extension of diaphragmatic breathing. You can do it any time and in any situation. First, find a comfortable place to sit back or lie down – a carpeted floor, a soft chair, a bed, or anywhere else you feel comfortable. Practice diaphragmatic breathing, as described in the previous section. Focus on taking slow, deep breaths that expand your entire chest. You might want to put your hands on your chest and stomach in the beginning. Focus your attention on the rise and fall of your stomach by actively watching each breath. After 10 or 20 guided diaphragmatic breaths, let each breath develop as it wishes. Follow each breath as it travels from your nostrils deep into your chest. Feel the rush of air from your lungs into your windpipe to your throat and out your nostrils. Watch your breaths as you might watch the waves on a seashore, slowly coming in and then going out again.

Often you will find that your thoughts, feelings, or daydreams disturb your focused breathing. Keep at it nonetheless. It is more important that you perform this exercise daily than it is that your technique be perfect. Visualization is never done perfectly. It is the journey, not the destination, that enables you to achieve long-term change. Continue to practice diaphragmatic breathing until you begin to feel relaxed. Once you are relaxed, your unconscious is ready to accept your visualization.

Visualizing is one way of focusing mental energy on a specific task. There is no right way to do it. Some people seem to sense someone moving around in a dark room. Others say that they just feel as if they are going over their goals. Still others consider visualization to be a thinking process, where they narrate to themselves each step of the story. So don't be concerned if you don't actively "see" your visualization. Just do the exercise and you will find your own way of getting results.

Spend five to ten minutes visualizing every day. You want to see yourself reaching your goals. Picture it as something really happening. You should spend a few minutes on your wellness image and a few minutes envisioning solutions to high-risk situations. We will provide more information on these subjects later in this chapter. Even if you can only manage five minutes during a break or sitting on a bus, be sure you do it. Experience in advance the rewards of your efforts and be grateful that you have the power to succeed. That way, you won't feel out of place when you do succeed.

Affirmations

During your daily visualization session, expressions of your growing unconscious sense of wellness will begin to occur to you. These may express themselves in images and words like beauty, liberation, freedom, choice, commitment, love, health, serenity, wholeness, cleansing, stability, co-operation, bliss, and calm. By writing down a few of these thoughts, you can help identify and strengthen this growing force within you. After a while, you should try to organize these words and thoughts into complete sentences to create your personalized wellness affirmation. An affirmation is a sentence or paragraph that summarizes your wellness goals. It is like the mission statement that many successful businesses use to focus their efforts. Most affirmations begin with "I am committed (or dedicated) to . . ." and end with ". . . each and every day." Until you develop your own affirmation and record it in your Wellness Planner, you can use this one:

> I am committed to promoting my health and achieving greater wellness each and every day.

You should say your affirmation, either out loud or silently, after each visualization. It punctuates and affirms your commitment to wellness. Many people also adopt a winning attitude to wellness by repeating their health affirmations at regular intervals every day.

Your Wellness Image

Many people have unrealistic or exaggerated mental images of how they will look and feel in the near future. This grandiose image of the new you is an overgeneralized picture in your mind that will inevitably leave you feeling unsatisfied. By overestimating your potential, you increase your risk of feeling helpless and hopeless, despite achieving significant gains. These negative thoughts activate your old friend, the Sedentary Slob. Defining a realistic wellness image will help you achieve success. Within your unconscious mind, your wellness image will become a reservoir of positive energy that you can then turn to wherever you feel uncertain about your new health commitments. Your daily visualization will be like a bank deposit that builds up your cash reserves for difficult times. You can draw on your wellness image in many different situations, which we will discuss in a later chapter.

Your wellness image is a movie clip of yourself in a specific situation that captures how you hope to look, feel, and be. To choose an image, focus on a time when you were striving toward a greater sense of physical well-being and succeeding. It might have been in high school, at the top of a ski lift, or after a great accomplishment. Focus on how good you felt about yourself.

Let us share with you an experience of how this technique can work. Here are two wellness images of one of the authors, Barry Simon.

Image #1: 1984

I'm riding my stationary bike, wearing a pair of wine-colored sweat pants, a Toronto T-shirt, running shoes, and white socks. Sweat is pouring down my face, as I push to hit the 35 m.p.h. mark on the speedometer. Bruce Springsteen is blasting through my earphones, pushing me to travel that extra mile.

My shoulders are pulled back, my chest is firm, and my stomach is flat, except for a small ridge of fat on the front of my gut, where my shirt is tucked into my pants. My thighs and calves are firm and well-defined. There is a satisfied smile on my face, and a sense of accomplishment, pride, and power runs through my body.

Notice that while my upper body is not "perfect", the image is in keeping with my first plateau of expected wellness. This visualization was a realistic, attainable image for me at the time. It focused my wellness desires for a year. Then, I began the annual process of redefining my goals and my wellness image.

After five years on the program, my wellness image had changed considerably:

Image #2: 1989

I'm wearing mirrored sunglasses, a black T-shirt, faded blue jeans, and high-cut jogging shoes that are splattered with pine needles from the forest floor. On my back is a knapsack filled with trail mix. Silently, I jog up the hill.

My pectoralis muscles outline my chest, my shoulders are firm, and there is (finally) a V-shape to my upper body! My stomach is mostly flat, but there is still a small area that gently bulges. My legs are firm and evenly developed. I feel a sense of calmness and serenity as I run up the hill. Reaching the top, I breathe deeply and smile. I look out on a still lake that reflects the surrounding mountains before me.

You can see that this image is tied to my own personality. It is quite different from my original visualization, but both reflect realistic, personal goals. The second image has a greater sense of holistic wellness that I could not have achieved without first successfully attaining four intermediate plateaus of change.

Now, it is your turn. Sit relaxed in a comfortable chair with a clipboard and pen on your lap. Then follow these steps to develop your wellness image.

1. Begin by imagining the setting – the background for your wellness image. It could be a room, a gym, a special beach, a skating rink, or a forest – your own fantasy land. Don't work too hard at it – just allow an image or thought to bubble up into your consciousness. Choose the image that seems to be the most harmonious with your goals. Open your eyes and briefly write down your wellness setting. Remember that the image will become more clear over the next few weeks, so don't rush the experience.

2. Next, imagine the body you are going to develop on the Winning Weigh program. Be reasonable! You are not ever going to look like Jane Fonda or Arnold Schwartzenegger if your basic skeletal structure and metabolism are different than theirs. Instead, commit yourself to developing the best possible *you.* Be specific. Become aware of your flexibility, the straightness of your back, your relaxed neck muscles, your expanded chest, your upper arms, your abdomen, and your hips. Really see your thighs, calves, and buttocks. Remember that bulges, tummies, and thighs are all part of being human. Imagine the clothes you would like to wear. Write down, in as much detail as you can, the physical aspects of your wellness body image.

3. Notice your facial expression. In your wellness image, carry your head high and smile with a glow of inner peace. Feel the energy and sense of wellness that radiates from you to the outside world. Emerson once said, "You can tell each man's sense of who he is by looking into his eyes." Imagine your eyes reflecting your new sense of inner direction and accomplishment.

4. Next, establish how you feel physically. Follow the lines of your chest and feel your chest expanding as you take slow, deep, revitalizing breaths. Notice the contour of your back. Get up and move around. Feel the flexibility and strength in your legs and the gentle bounce in your walk that symbolize a new healthy you. Feel your muscle tone, your body's flexibility, your slowed heart beat, and your fresh skin. Feel the sense of wellness when your body is in top physical shape.

5. Finally, imagine your emotions when you achieve your wellness goals. Imagine what you will think. Make a list of the words, phrases, and thoughts that capture the new you: alive, serene, joyous, directed, committed, sensual, centered. Write some affirmations about how good you feel.

6. Collect all these separate images, put them together, and create a unified, synthesized wellness image. It is very important to set an attainable image. Be reasonable! Remember that you will reset your wellness images as you attain your goals. If part of the image makes you feel anxious, then stop and make sure it's realistic. On the other hand, a little anxiety may be excitement at the prospect of change.

High-Risk Situations

A high-risk situation is any circumstance in which you have repeatedly made disease-promoting decisions in the past. Look back at your list of Sedentary Slob activators. These will give you an idea of some of your high-risk situations. They might include a tradition of a late-night snack or an after-work drink, being bored at home, feeling lonely, late afternoon fatigue, escalating hunger while watching TV, or being too busy to exercise. Using visualization, you can create mental videos of yourself overcoming these high-risk situations. These visualizations will create new neural pathways that will help you succeed in a real crisis. You will begin to convince your unconscious mind that you are destined to succeed. This positive memory will energize and guide your actions when you face the challenge of actual high-risk situations. You should always have enough details to make the situation seem completely real.

Here's an example of a visualization used by one of our patients to deal with a high-risk situation:

> I am sitting on the couch, watching TV. I become bored, so I get up and calmly walk into the kitchen. I pour a tall glass of mineral water and squeeze in a lime. My inner sense of peacefulness and directness makes me stand tall and walk with confidence.

Every day, after you have visualized your wellness image and repeated your wellness affirmation, start visualizing your high-risk situation. See yourself carrying out the solution to your obstacle perfectly and with confidence. Remember that you don't actually need to *see* the image – just focus your energy on carrying out the solution perfectly in your imagination. In slow motion, see, think, and feel yourself making the moves that will guarantee success. Focus on the positive sense of accomplishment that glows on your face and in your eyes. Feel the power, strength, and ease with which you achieve your goals. Experience the pleasure, joy, and excitement of success.

End the high-risk visualization by returning to your wellness image. Repeat your wellness affirmation and then return your attention to your breathing for another 60 seconds before opening your eyes. The extra time you spend in a relaxed state will deepen and strengthen your unconscious wellness image.

This simple exercise, repeated regularly, is crucial to overcoming your tendencies to abandon your good resolutions. Most people have five or six typical high-risk situations. By rotating them, you can go through them all in one week.

In time, you will energize new challenges and opportunities through visualization. Many athletes, performers, and businesspeople use visualization to prepare for the uncertainties and challenges of our high-speed competitive worlds.

Starting Right Now . . .

1. Begin practicing diaphragmatic breathing for five to ten minutes each day.

2. When you feel anxious or under stress during the day, take several deep diaphragmatic breaths and notice the changes you feel.

3. Spend five minutes daily for two weeks defining and modifying your wellness image. Once you have a well-defined wellness image, write it down in the Wellness Planner.

4. Write down any words or thoughts that come to mind during your visualization sessions and develop your own wellness affirmations. Write them down in the Wellness Planner (p. 321). Repeat your affirmation after each visualization session and regularly during the day.

5. Turn back to your list of Sedentary Slob activators. Create a solution for each – a personalized specific, step-by-step plan for overcoming your activator. Develop a visualization for each activator in which you see yourself carrying out the solution. In the Wellness Planner (p. 322), write a detailed description, including the setting, the time of day, and the specific circumstances.

6. Take five to ten minutes every day to visualize using this simple routine:

    a. After getting comfortable, practice diaphragmatic breathing until you are relaxed.
    b. Visualize your wellness image for at least two minutes.
    c. Say your wellness affirmation silently or out loud.
    d. Visualize the solution to one or more of your high-risk situations.
    e. Repeat your wellness affirmation.
    f. Focus on your diaphragmatic breathing for another 30 seconds before opening your eyes.

Summary for Step 5

1. Your unconscious mind is a collection of your lifetime experiences, memories, thoughts, and emotions.

2. Your unconscious lifestyle script includes three distinct acts:
   Act I: The Blissful Binge

Act II: The Perfect Forever Fantasy
Act III: The Revolution

3. Watch out for the three main activators: situations, people, and energy states that awaken your Sedentary Slob.

4. Look to the outline on pages 204-205 to see how to change your thinking style.

5. Breathing and posturizing are two helpful ways to adopt a winning attitude.

6. By using visualization you can begin to develop a realistic wellness image. By adding your own version of an affirmation you can punctuate your wellness image.

7. Allow yourself to develop a series of wellness images and strategies for high-risk situations.

8. Begin to see yourself as shifting out on your Sedentary Slob and into your new wellness image.

STEP 6   LIVING IN THE MOMENT

In everyday life, little decisions just don't feel that urgent. It's hard to see the consideration of whether to have a chocolate bar after lunch as a life-or-death decision. And yet the accumulation of such minor choices can end your life prematurely through cancer, heart attack, or a stroke. You have to balance the long-term benefits against the moment of temptation. That's why it's important for you to develop a long-term perspective on your health. Rarely does it seem urgent that you do a particular exercise or look for a high-fiber breakfast on a given morning, but all these in-the-moment decisions contribute to meeting your long-term goals.

We have been through the process ourselves, and we have been helping others for a long time. We understand the difficulties that you will have in making wellness choices every day. Often your best intentions can be completely sabotaged by a friend who arrives at your home bearing a dozen doughnuts or an ice cream cake. Perhaps you're overtaken by the festive spirit at a wedding or party or bored at a company banquet. In all these scenarios, you're trying to stick to your wellness plans but are caught up in the moment and vulnerable to temptation. Situations like these will occur all your life. And although you will give in sometimes, you need to acquire techniques for making less damaging choices. As long as you believe your goals are worthwhile and you're willing to work to accomplish them, you can ultimately change your bad habits to wellness habits.

Playful and Powerful
To succeed on the Winning Weigh program, learn to say to yourself, "I might have been this way for ten years, but in this moment I truly have the opportunity to change." On many health promotion programs, you only need to obey the letter of the law that the program lays down. If it says to have a breast of chicken on Thursday for lunch, you do just that. We believe that this obedience makes you feel passive, weak, and submissive to the program. From that position,

any failure or setback on the program is seen as one more example of your lifelong inadequacies. It's not long before your weak and passive feelings lead you off into a blissful binge and another cycle of disease-promoting behavior.

Don't fall into the trap of believing that you need to follow orders slavishly in order to succeed. The secret to living in the moment is seeing your ability to change. That means that every exercise will only be beneficial if you approach it with the intent to make it work for you. Make your choices with knowledge, conviction, and dedication.

If you agree to perform each exercise with the certainty that you will be one more success story, then you will be on the way to being an independent agent of your own wellness. We will give you advice, but you can only accomplish things on your own. For most people, that is a frightening thought. People often prefer to be given the one right answer, or, better yet, have someone else just do it for them.

Forget about a knight in shining armour coming along and rescuing you from yourself. You need to make a critical shift in your thinking. It is time to begin awakening the sleeping giant within yourself.

We cannot tell you exactly what you should eat, how much food you'll need, or what your realistic weight range will be. We can suggest general exercise plans, but we can't predict how soothing exercise or meditation will be for you. In this same way, we cannot predict which in-the-moment techniques will be most effective for you. A program that will work for you for a lifetime must be your plan. Your version of the Winning Weigh plan will come from experimenting and playing with the many possible methods we suggest. We truly mean *play*, because it will take weeks and, in some cases, months to arrive at a combination that will work for you in a variety of situations.

If you continue to feel submissive and obedient, you will never succeed. To find your personal wellness plan, you will need to recognize your own strength. Make use of your power to pause and assess. You have the power to make a new choice.

Most of the exercises in this section of the book are designed to make you stop and say "I can be powerful" and "I can change." But don't take yourself too seriously. We don't want you developing a furrowed brow and a serious look as you perform the exercises in this book. If you are too serious and intense, each small setback (and we all experience setbacks) will seem to be a giant failure.

So be playful! One of the best ways to lock into this fun-loving approach is to smile and roll your shoulders back. By smiling and recognizing your ability to actively commit to wellness, you will begin to approach each situation with the idea that "this moment is the only moment that really counts. I can choose to be the old me or I can commit myself to the change I desire."

What Is "Living in the Moment"?

Step 6 is about changing, about becoming different than you were a moment ago. Change is not a lifetime plan, a promise to be perfect forever. It is a challenge that you will face each moment of your life.

The only time you can make a decision to change is in the current moment. Only if you focus on this very moment instead of on the past or future, can you alter your habits, regardless of how much reading, planning, and visualizing you do. In each moment of your lifetime, you make either a health-promoting or a disease-promoting choice. With each health-promoting choice, you take one step in a shift toward wellness – you begin to take active control of your health, your body, and your life.

To begin this shift, slow down the film and start looking at your life one frame at a time, one moment and one choice at a time. Slowing down will allow you to become conscious of your automatic behavior as you do what your Sedentary Slob or Self-Righteous Snob script dictates. You have to accept that you are human, with strengths and weaknesses. You will have the odd disease-promoting food simply because it provides immediate pleasure. The Winning Weigh isn't about being perfect; it's about undoing some of your automatic patterns of eating and exercising so you can increase the number of health-promoting decisions you make.

Intensity Levels

Your capacity to make health-promoting decisions probably varies. Sometimes, you are so enthusiastic that you make wellness choices easily At other times, you are so frustrated that you feel you may act on your disease-promoting urges in stubborn rebellion. Then, there are times when you may happily indulge in disease-promoting decisions. We call these three ways of feeling ***intensity levels.*** Most of the day, you won't need to consider which level of intensity you are in, but when you are faced with a wellness choice, you will have more control of the situation if you understand how these intensity levels affect your ability to choose wisely. Let's look at these three ways of feeling and thinking.

1. Overwhelming Intensity

During periods of overwhelming intensity, your feelings are very strong. You might feel tired, sad, anxious, angry, or frustrated, and your reaction is to act out a typical Sedentary Slob pattern of behavior. You might skip a workout, eat a big bowl of ice cream, or simply sit home and sulk. Don't confuse this behavior with making a conscious disease-promoting *choice* because you need a night off. In an overwhelming intensity state, you are too overwhelmed to make real choices; you end up following your automatic script as a way out of your emotional dilemma.

2. Optimum Intensity

During periods of optimum intensity, you can make choices with little regret or difficulty. You can quickly assess the situation and make either a health-promoting or disease-promoting decision. If you felt this way all the time, you would have no need for the Winning Weigh program.

3. Insufficient Intensity

In a state of insufficient intensity, you simply do, with no regard for the consequences. This state differs from optimum intensity in that you omit the critical step of assessing the options. In terms of wellness, you ignore the needs and susceptibilities of your body. Insufficient intensity is *comfort zone* living. That's when you lie on the couch, beer in one hand, chips in the other, watching television instead of participating actively in life. In this intensity, there are no automatic Sedentary Slob thinking styles or any feelings of fear or sadness. You simply do what you want to do, with no regard for your body or health.

Intensity levels are your link to living in the moment. Ultimately, whether you succeed in a moment or not is dependent on how you feel and how motivated you are. These qualities will be influenced by the level of anxiety you feel.

Anxiety is not always severe enough to register on your consciousness, but it does influence your behavior. High anxiety will sweep you away, out of control, creating the state we refer to as overwhelming intensity. On the other extreme, if you are feeling no particular anxiety, you will have no motivation to make careful choices or to change your characteristic behavior patterns.

Your Internal Director

To be able to label your intensity levels, we must first enhance your ability to identify your intensity level. To do this, we'd like to introduce you to your Internal Director. Think of your lifestyle script as a play and your Sedentary Slob as the role you automatically play, over and over again. To stop this repeating story line, you need a director to yell "Cut!"

Your Internal Director watches you experience life. If you can see events from that point of view, you'll begin to witness your thoughts, feelings, and actions as an outsider would see them. As we discussed earlier, most people play roles in their lifestyle scripts with little thought about the consequences and little awareness of the plot. In terms of wellness, they often switch back and forth between the Sedentary Slob and the Self-Righteous Snob without realizing that both parts are dead ends. If you empower your Internal Director, you can change this automatic script.

One of the best ways to get in touch with your Internal Director is through the diaphragmatic breathing described in the visualization chapter. Start diaphragmatic breathing now. Concentrate on your nostrils as air comes in and out. Your ability to watch yourself breathe is your Internal Director. The part of your mind that just asked "Am I doing it right?" is also your Internal Director. Many people experience their Internal Director as a mind-space behind their eyes that watches as they play out their parts. Sometimes the Internal Director seems to be missing the performance. Diaphragmatic breathing increases your level of awareness and brings the Internal Director to center stage.

By stepping back from the action, you give your Internal Director the opportunity to guide your actions. We call this the *freeze frame*. It is the moment in the script when your Internal Director sees how the scene is shaping up, where the different roles are, and what mood is being created.

If you have never consciously turned to your Internal Director, you'll need to develop a technique for doing that. Your goal is to create a freeze frame in which to make a new choice. Creating such moments gives you an opportunity to bring about long-term change. When you recognize a moment in which you have an opportunity to make a wellness choice, follow the procedure. Like practicing your scales when learning to play the piano, the exercise might seem burdensome, but following it is critical to your success.

1. Take three deep diaphragmatic breaths. Watch for your increased awareness as your Internal Director's space appears behind your eyes. This is a subtle shift, so don't take an all-or-nothing attitude toward it.
2. If you are standing, take two steps backwards, ending up with your feet together. If you are sitting, bring your hands together in a prayer position on your lap.
3. Take a couple more deep breaths as you assess your intensity level.

Let's look at this process in action. You are at a wedding. You're feeling good, having just enjoyed a healthy dinner and some dancing. Then they bring out the desserts. Walking toward the table, you notice that you are becoming increasingly anxious and excited. You recognize the approach of an overwhelming intensity moment. This is an opportunity for taking control of your actions.

JB, one of our patients, had an ongoing battle with her desire for sweets. She often found herself in this situation, and she would end up eating large mounds of desserts without really enjoying them. By using diaphragmatic breathing, we taught her to enter her Internal Director's space. She could then step back from the table and temporarily short-circuit her automatic script. By taking the slow deep breaths, she experienced a calmness instead of the overwhelming intensity that was in keeping with this script. She found it easier and easier to avoid gorging on sweets.

People we have worked with are demoralized and troubled by the number of diets and programs they've tried. You will be surprised how just a simple shift in your intensity level will greatly affect your chances of success. Many of our patients have said, "Why bother with this Internal Director stuff?" or "It didn't work the first time, so why try it for a whole month?" All of your failures and setbacks have put you at the risk of seeing yourself as a lost cause. Just remember – whether you say you can or you can't, you're right.

This habit of stepping back becomes more ingrained as you practice. Much like learning to ride a bike, you first need to get your balance. However, once you get it, you will have it for the rest of your life. For many people, turning to the Internal Director is awkward the first hundred times, but it does eventually become automatic. Keep that in mind as you try out these techniques. In the following chapters, we will look at some specific ways to switch out of an overwhelming intensity level and an insufficient intensity level.

Exhibit 6–1
Intensity Levels

Overwhelming Intensity

- The intensity is so great that you feel unable to act out the choice you have made.

- Your unconscious mind automatically follows a pattern of behavior that it has been programmed to follow in similar situations in the past.

Optimum Intensity

- You feel calm yet motivated to carry out your conscious choices.

Insufficient Intensity
- Both your intensity and your motivation levels are very low.
- You are content to remain in your comfort zone and to follow your automatic behavior.

Making a 15-Minute Commitment

How good is your record at carrying out New Year's resolutions? Do you find yourself reluctant to make resolutions anymore? Conscious change is frightening when you feel it is final and absolute. If you use words like "never," "forever," and "always," you increase the pressure on yourself. In the end, you feel resentment, anger, and disappointment with your goals and with yourself.

On the Winning Weigh program, we advise you to start with 15-minute commitments to your wellness goals. These short-term commitments guarantee that you do not make any resolutions you don't feel you can achieve. This pattern will decrease your nervousness about committing to act in a health-promoting way. You'll avoid the fear that you'll be anxious forever. Every time you meet one of these bite-sized commitments, you are building a foundation of successful wellness-oriented experiences. You will see your beliefs about yourself change, while you protect yourself from feeling overcontrolled. You will confirm your ability to make choices.

In many cases, anxious feelings pass quickly and in just 15 minutes you find yourself in a different state of mind. Once you gain trust and confidence with the 15-minute commitment, you can expand to a 30-minute commitment. Eventually you may get to the point where you are making day-long commitments.

Action: Empowering Your Wellness Role

Making and keeping a commitment, even for 15 minutes, means taking self-directed action. The British poet Lord Alfred Tennyson once wrote, "I must lose myself in action, lest I wither in despair." Action has the power to shift you from a passive, helpless role into a motivated, enthusiastic one. Any time you actively combine a 15-minute commitment with action, you inevitably begin to develop new beliefs about yourself. No action is too small to help bring about this shift.

It is your ability to guide and modify your future that is forgotten in a state of overwheming or insufficient intensity. Each time you stop, adjust the level of intensity, and make a wellness choice, you have done something important, but it will only contribute to your health if it ends with a direct action.

To make your actions effective, we have three suggestions:

1. Exaggerate every action.

Since a part of you is helpless and waiting to be taken care of, you need to reawaken your own sleeping giant. To do this, you need to use your body/mind linkage. Each time you step back into the director's chair, do it with a great deal of physical intensity. Step back quickly and with certainty. If you are sitting, bring your hands together quickly and with conviction. Take deep breaths, and feel your chest expanding. Raise your head and look up as you breathe inwards.

Slow, passive movements will leave you in a weakened, passive attitude. Do it right! Force yourself to be in the moment! Seize this moment and be the best possible you!

Make each 15-minute commitment an active choice. Decide to walk away from the table without dessert, and then do it briskly, your head held high and a smile on your face. Once having made a commitment, carry it out with dedication and power. Each time you make a 15-minute commitment and choose an action, ask yourself, "Am I carrying this out in a physically committed way? Am I playful and powerful in this moment? Can I emphasize my conviction by physically acting in a more definite, committed way?" Remember that in every moment your physical commitment can either amplify or nullify your ability to be playful and powerful.

2. Start Small

Begin by choosing to make a small but firm change in your life. The old saying "Don't bite off more then you can chew" reflects the need to define goals that are achievable.

3. Just Do It!

This slogan works well for Nike sports shoes, because it is what exercise and motion is all about. Just do it! You may have doubts and uncertainties, you can't be sure how it will work out, but you just step in and do it anyway. And do it now!

The critical ingredient to completing your wellness shift lies in actually making a choice and acting on it. The very act of doing something in the outside world pulls you out of your Sedentary Slob into your Internal Director's chair and into a brand new state of mind. Action is the most powerful acknowledgement of your ability to make a choice. Every time you make a commitment and perform an action consistent with that commitment, you reactivate your sense of inner strength and self-direction.

William James, in **Principles of Psychology**, wrote, "Where indecision is great, before a giant leap, consciousness is agonizingly intense." When you commit yourself to stepping out of your Sedentary Slob role and following your new wellness approach, your anxiety and nervousness *will* increase. This is inevitable because you are contradicting your well-ingrained patterns of behavior. Remember that your unconscious has no concept of better or worse, just an automatic program showing what is and what is not part of your typical behavior. So whenever you first try to change your behavior, you will feel threatened.

This threatened feeling comes from your unconscious mind, which sets off an alarm that says, "Hey, what you're about to do goes against my game plan!" Your unconscious sees your new ideas about wellness as intruders. Suddenly, you are faced with a conflict – either remain the way you've been or choose the wellness option. To your unconscious, your conflict between your Sedentary Slob and your new wellness role is not based on a choice between right and wrong. It is based on a choice of remaining in your current, comfortable, automatic script or breaking into a new and challenging way of living.

This moment of indecision is called a *crisis*. In Japanese, the word *crisis* has two symbols: one represents danger and the other represents opportunity. Every opportunity for change is bound to be perceived as dangerous. Your feelings of uncertainty and nervousness are reminders of the potentially giant leap that you are about to make. With time, however, you will begin to make health-promoting decisions automatically.

All the techniques in the Winning Weigh program – including the eating plan, exercise programs, goal-setting techniques, and visualization exercises – are designed to encourage a health-promoting choice in the moment. So begin to make each moment – whether a moment of overwhelming intensity or insufficient intensity – an opportunity to succeed at wellness through your actions. After you've acted, see how you feel about your decision. Only by objectively reviewing your choices can you modify your future behavior. Don't waste energy blaming yourself if you make a disease-promoting choice this time. Instead, see every choice as an opportunity to evaluate the pleasure you derived from the immediate benefit.

Starting Right Now . . .

When you recognize a moment in which you have an opportunity to make a wellness choice, create a freeze frame so you can make a conscious choice by following these steps:

1. Take three deep diaphragmatic breaths. Watch for your increased awareness as your Internal Director's space appears behind your eyes.
2. If you are standing, take two steps backwards, ending up with your feet together. If you are sitting, bring your hands together in a prayer position on your lap.
3. Take a couple more deep breaths as you assess your intensity level.

Shifting Out of Overwhelming Intensity

Overwhelming intensity makes you feel helpless and anxious. Because you feel unable to make choices, you take the simplest route, doing things the way you have always done them before. Does the following pattern of behavior sound familiar?

It was 11:15 at night. Lynne was sitting alone in her apartment watching the evening news when the telephone rang. Glad to get a call from anyone on this boring evening, she picked up the receiver with anticipation only to find that the line was dead. She was left discontented and a little lonely. A commercial for ice cream came on television, and suddenly ice cream seemed like a good idea, even though she had promised herself to start eating only healthful foods. Dutifully, she stayed by the screen until the news came back on. A town had been destroyed by an earthquake. With people dying in earthquakes, boycotting ice cream didn't seem worthwhile.

On the fridge door was a warning sign: "Trespassers after 10:00 will be prosecuted." Lynne had put it there to guard against her own weakness. Now, she was torn between the urge to be strong and the urge to be self-indulgent. No contest. She dished out a huge bowl of ice cream and wolfed it down while standing in the kitchen. As the ice cream disappeared, her shame at her own lack of discipline grew.

This example captures many of the characteristics of an overwhelming intensity moment. Lynne felt drawn to the refrigerator because she was reaching the blissful binge part of her lifestyle script. She dished out the ice cream automatically, having reverted to her familiar Sedentary Slob role. The situation had certain activators (the late hour, the telephone call, the depressing newscast). It was also closely connected to anxiety.

You may have started eating some wellness-promoting foods, have learned some relaxation techniques, or be on a regular exercise program but still not recognize your own version of overwhelming intensity. That's because you have reached a plateau of change, and you work within that boundary of health promotion. Each time you venture beyond that boundary, whether it is towards greater health or away from it, you probably experience a sense of anxiety. This tension may be subtle, but it still has a definite impact on your psychological make-up.

Typically, your body gets used to receiving a certain percentage of fat from your diet or following a particular exercise regimen each day. If you attempt to change this pattern, you will experience a sense of uneasiness. If you aren't paying attention, this anxiety will be missed, because it will quickly be followed by an automatic choice that is within the boundary you have set for yourself.

A marathon runner we worked with described his experience of overwhelming intensity. He was out for a Chinese dinner and chose the non-greasy, broccoli-rich dish moo goo guy pan. But as he was about to order, he suddenly felt tense because he knew he wouldn't be enjoying his favorite chicken-fried rice. This was followed by a sense of sadness and a knotting in his stomach as he struggled to decide.

The critical aspect of this example is the subtle, conscious experience of fear and regret. Those feelings were a mild, but significant version of the overwhelming intensity state. All these feelings have the power to sway you to choose your customary route. The unconscious searches for the least tension-producing behavior, and that is the one most commomly chosen.

An overwhelming intensity has three typical steps:

1. You are in a completely overwhelmed state like Lynne (our first example) and regret does not occur until after the disease-promoting choice has been made. Or, like our marathon runner, there is a recognition of a moment of potential change, which inevitably induces a moment of psychological overwhelming intensity.

2. During this moment of potential change, you feel unsure, tense, even sad, because you are aware that you have a choice.

3. This awareness is followed by behavior that is in keeping with your typical lifestyle pattern. You need to struggle with

your own version of overwhelming intensity before you will be able to break that distant barrier.

Certain situations, emotions, thoughts, and bodily feelings will be linked to your overwhelming intensity state. Here are some more examples of common overwhelming intensity situations that have been described to us.

The late afternoon is the toughest time of day for me. Dizzy, tired, hit by a wave of weakness, I rush to the store downstairs for a chocolate bar. Hurrying back to my office, I feel tense and guilty for eating another 450-calorie time bomb.

I usually make dinner for five other people. Being around all that food from five o'clock onward, I just automatically taste everything. I feel partially full by the time I sit down for the meal and get angry at myself for having eaten so much, but that just seems to make me pig out all the more at the table. I always seem to end up blaming myself for being so weak and making false promises to be stronger tomorrow.

Whenever I go out with some guy I really like and he doesn't call me back the next day, I just seem to need to fill up on treats. I'll eat partially frozen freezer cakes, big plates of creamy pasta, and almost anything else. I even start smoking again.
I just feel "What's the use? I'll never find somebody to love."

The guys have been getting together to play cards every Thursday for five years. Bob always has both fruit salad and his famous buttercup cookies available. Well, after a bowl of fruit salad, I get this elusive feeling that I'm missing something and that everyone else is having more fun. Quickly, I gulp down a cookie or two. I often realize that they aren't as good as I had remembered them, but I can't seem to break the pattern.

Every weekend I'd run five, maybe six miles. One weekend I ran ten miles and, from that point on, I steadily increased my distance. Getting beyond the the ten-mile-point was a real challenge. Each time I started to go the extra mile, I began to fear that something bad would happen to my body or that I would fail. For no rational reason, I'd suddenly feel tired, weak, and in need of turning back.

You'd think I get a tapeworm with my period. I eat constantly and I am sensitive to everyone's criticisms and comments. The day I finish my period, that little tapeworm goes back to sleep, and I get started trying to take off the two pounds I've gained during the week.

Vacations give me permission to cheat on my normal diet. When I'm on vacation, I'm drawn to every fast-food restaurant I pass. I'm a street vendor's dream. I sometimes wonder if they have my picture hanging in their carts as "Customer of the Month." It takes me three weeks to get back on track after a two-week vacation. Just mentioning the word "vacation" gets my taste buds working overtime.

Each of these events is an example of overwhelming intensity because it begins with some outside stimulus that creates the opportunity to claim that what happens next is not really under the control of the person in the situation.

Switching out of an overwhelming intensity style is not easy. To begin to change, you first need to recognize that you are in an overwhelming intensity moment. You have already identified your Sedentary Slob activators (early in Step 5), and they should warn you of an impending overwhelming intensity crisis. You might feel anxious, fearful, sad, or out of control. You might be using one of the ten thinking styles we looked at in Step 5. Your body feels nervous. Perhaps there is a tightness in your face, cramps in your stomach, or a closed feeling in your chest that is keeping you from breathing easily. Your shoulders will tend to be rounded, your head sunk in your neck, and your face frowning. You are about to act in a way that is not quite within your own free will. You will feel as though you're acting out a script for a character you don't want to play.

Many times, as we have stressed, it is only a simple wave of nervousness about your ability to succeed or regret about the loss of your favorite food that will shift you into your standard, rigid pattern. An overwhelming state occurs any time you think about a wellness oppurtunity and then begin to feel signs of anxiety – a tension in your throat, butterflies in your stomach, a feeling of sadness, or any apprehension about your new choice. It is these subtle shifts, in addition to the panic moments, that guide you in the moments when opportunities to change arise.

When you find yourself near or in an overwhelming intensity state, carry out the actions you learned in the last chapter:

1. Do your diaphragmatic breathing.
2. Step back to get to your Internal Director's chair.
3. Freeze the frame.
4. Break out of the old script by seeing your way out, thinking your way out, talking your way out, or acting your way out. (We'll go through this group of techniques in detail in the pages that follow.)

When we first teach these steps to people, they typically become overwhelmed. Don't give in to the overwhelmed state by saying to yourself "I can't use all these techniques." Instead, read our instructions carefully. Try them one at a time. Then, reread the instructions to make sure you have them right. Once you have tried following our recommended procedures a few times in your daily life, try experimenting with them a little. Like a scientist looking for the right formula, you may try several combinations before you find the technique that works right for you. Once you have discovered your formula, use it every time you are in an overwhelming moment. You can change only through practice. By sticking with it, you can increase your sense of power and choice.

Seeing Your Way Out

In the visualization section of Step 5, we stressed the importance of developing a wellness image. Your wellness image is a healthy, attainable image of yourself. Through regular practice, you should have given this image a calm, relaxed aura. When you are anxious and overwhelmed, you need to contact this calm, committed self. As you find ourself drawn into a disease-promoting activity by overwhelming intensity, step back, sit in your Internal Director's chair, and bring your wellness image into focus. This image will break your automatic link to your lifestyle script. The more often you practice visualizing your wellness image, the more power it will have to calm and direct you.

Greg, a senior executive at a major corporation, found that he'd have the urge to order a hamburger and fries to eat at his desk while working. Initially resisting, he'd feel a sense of sadness and regret as he ordered the vegetable platter and chicken breast sandwich. Giving in to this tension, he'd call back and change his order. He would then feel ashamed but satisfied with his burger and fries. After learning to recognize the mild apprehension he experienced in this situation, Greg would simply begin his deep breathing, press his hands together firmly, and bring his wellness image to mind. He continued to take slow, deep breaths, focusing on the image, until his food arrived. Smiling playfully and powerfully, his wellness image still strong in his mind, he dug into his meal. By doing this over and over, Greg was able to develop his wellness image and use it whenever he ordered food, thereby taking an active control over this important aspect of his life.

Thinking Your Way Out

You can also ***think*** your way out of overwhelming intensity states. How would you deal with the following situation?

It's 5:30 p.m. and you have a dinner date with Barbara at 7:00. You tell yourself, "I'd love to go for a run, but I don't have time. Boy, I really resent Barb for expecting me to be so punctual [blaming others]. Of course, if I had finished my work earlier I would have had time [blaming yourself]. You spend the evening feeling angry and frustrated.

What identifies this scene as an overwhelming intensity moment is that you feel unable to break out of the situation. The thinking pattern illustrated here has been developed to justify following your lifestyle script. By listening to yourself and labelling the thinking styles you use (as we did in brackets in the passage above), you can learn to step back and solve problems in a new way. You can recognize that this is one way of thinking but it is not necessarily the only way. Maybe you could go for a short run. Maybe you could see if Barb would accept your arriving 20 minutes late. Maybe Barb wants to work out too. Explore other options rather than acting blindly.

Remember that your thinking style affects your behavior directly and it also affects how you feel. When you are angry because you are blaming others or frustrated because you are blaming yourself, you are more likely to indulge in self-indulgent, disease-promoting behavior.

Rewriting the Script

For some people, simply recognizing the thinking styles creates enough emotional distance from the lifestyle script to permit a change. Most of us need to practice in order to learn to rewrite the script.

Rewriting your script simply means that you no longer accept unconsciously playing out the same monologue, performance after performance. Instead, you begin to question and creatively shift the script you have accepted for years. Your script will be well established by now and it will have a typical monologue. Nonetheless, rewriting your script can be as easy as ABC. Let's take a look at the method.

A: Examine your thoughts to identify your thinking styles.

The first step requires you to learn to monitor the constant flow of thoughts in your mind. You need to identify those thoughts that reinforce the patterns you are trying to break. For example, you eat a plate of french fries and you have the thought, "I know I should not be eating these fries. I am so weak. I'll never get myself to follow a healthy diet." To recognize such thoughts, you need to step back for perspective. That's why we have shown you how to find your Internal Director's chair. Look at your thoughts from there.

When you have found such thoughts, label them. You already have a list of ten common thinking styles, and you will probably come up with a few more of your own. Start collecting them on either 3" x 5" cards or in a small notebook. Draw two columns. List the thought in the first column and label the thinking style in the second.

Thought	**Thinking style**
I am so weak. I'll never get myself to follow a healthy diet.	weak and dizzy; feeling forecasting

You will be amazed at how often thoughts repeat themselves and then guide how you act and feel.

Let's try a situation that is familiar to many people:

> I want to go to the gym, but I feel too tired. I can't decide whether to go or not. Why am I always pushing myself? Why can't I ever relax?

How do you feel reading that over? Does it ever happen to you? You rarely go home and feel relaxed after a monologue like that. Instead, you will typically feel weak and uncertain about what to do next.

B: Devise alternative ways of looking at a situation.
By having played in 500 performances of your lifestyle script, you begin to regard your script as unchangeable reality. By becoming aware of alternative ways of handling a situation, you can then see new scenerios.

You may suffer from the "Dagwood syndrome," the irresistable temptation to get out of bed at night and build a large sandwich for yourself. You should find out if the urge really is resistable. Try waiting 30 seconds before moving out of bed to establish your power over the situation. Try standing on one foot in front of the refrigerator for 15 seconds to prove to that you are actually making decisions.

The oddest actions are sometimes ascribed to weakness. One woman called herself weak and dizzy when she gave in to the urge for a Danish pastry. Travelling five blocks out of her way, she parked illegally while going to the bank machine. While eating the pastry, she still had the thought "I'm so weak." Yet she had made a considerable active effort to indulge her whim.

Blaming yourself assumes that you've made some error, and it somehow gets you out of asking critical questions like, "What can I do differently the next time I'm in a similar situation?" or "How does blaming myself affect my ability to solve my problem?" Blaming yourself allows you to give up on the situation.

If you find that you are blaming yourself for the sins you are about to commit, you could stop and ask, "Am I blowing this whole experience out of proportion?" Think how easy it would really be to drive past that fast-food restaurant or to make time for a workout at the gym or a walk.

Do you ever catch yourself feeling resentful that the hosts at the party you are attending are sabotaging your wellness program by serving your favorite sinful foods? What do you get out of being angry with the hosts? (You found someone else to blame, perhaps?) All too often people use such emotions to give themselves permission to eat food they know they should avoid. Ask yourself some questions about such emotions. What are the chances that my hosts know about my new attitudes? Just because food is there, do I really have to eat it?

Learn to develop substitutes. Look around the table for options; foods like fruit salad can keep you away from pastries. Look for non-food substitutes as well: see if there is someone you'd like to speak to instead of lingering near the buffet table while desserts are being brought out. A hug can be a good alternative to eating a comforting food.

How often have you skipped a workout because you are too tired to go the club to exercise? You may be too tired at that moment to see yourself doing your full workout, but could you manage a walk or a short run? Would you feel more motivated by a game of tennis or a swim? Ask yourself such questions to confront **all-or-nothing thinking.** You are using all-or-nothing thinking when you say "It's my usual way, and if I can't do that I might as well forget the whole thing." Train your Internal Director to recognize this pattern of thinking and learn to ask the questions that will open up other options. Once you are actually in the exercise situation and working out that feeling of overwhelming intensity will dissolve.

Once you are aware of alternative ways of thinking about a situation, you can choose to act differently. Through your actions, you can learn more about yourself, so that you will not necessarily be locked into one repetitive way of thinking.

Maybe you aren't going to your workout because you think you'll be too tired afterward. You are using the thinking style we have labelled "feeling forecasting." You anticipate how you will feel in the future, or you assume that your present feeling will be around forever.

Try to counter this pattern of thinking by gathering empirical data about yourself. Go to the gym for your workout anyway. Before you leave for the gym, predict in writing how you will feel after your workout. When you have finished your workout, make another entry about how you feel then. Be specific. Using a scale of one to five, assign an overall score to your sense of well-being. Be formal: try using a form like Exhibit 6-2 to track your feelings.

Exhibit 6–2
Forecast of How I Will Feel after Exercising

BEFORE (scale of 1 to 5):
AFTER (scale of 1 to 5):

By comparing your forecast with the actual event, you may find that you feel much better after a workout than you predicted you would. You can use the same method for any health-promoting activity (hiking, biking, long walks in the fall).

Some people use a note describing how they feel in more detail. A typical note might cover your thoughts, feelings, sense of well-being, energy level, and body image. One patient wrote the following note about how she felt after an exercise session:

> Great! Light, happy, silly, light as a feather! A smile on my face, a calmness in my body, and a sense of it being great to be alive!

Certainly this kind of enthusiasm doesn't follow every workout, but when it does, capturing it on paper may be a good idea. That note can be a very powerful motivator if you pull it out of your wallet and read it when you are trying to decide whether to go to the gym.

Summary: Typical questions you can ask yourself when in a situation of overwhelming intensity are:

1. What are two or three reasons why the way I'm thinking about this situation is not appropriate?
2. Am I confusing a thought with reality?
3. Are there other ways to look at this situation?
4. How can I test the thinking style I am using?
5. Can I act differently by being playful and powerful?

C: Consider the actual worst-case scenerio.
A single event can sometimes take on an overwhelming intensity. If you cannot help but do something you know you shouldn't do, at least try to free yourself from unnecessary anxiety and tension. To help decrease your fear, you can ask yourself, "What would be the effect of giving into this wish or fear?" What are the long-term effects of having candy one time this week? What will happen if I take the day off from my exercise routine? Try the following test.

1. Rate how fearful you are that you are about to act on your thought. Use a 1-to-5 scale. You can rate fear by how nervous you feel, your sense of helplessness, how weak you feel, the butterflies in your stomach, or the sense that you are about to act and can't change that from happening.

2. Ask yourself what the real implications of this action are. To answer that question simply look at what you want to do and see how this would fit into your over-all assessment of your health-promoting attitude. Would one or two cookies ruin your entire week? Is there a compromise food, like low-fat soft ice cream or gelato instead of the very creamy type? Could you accept a compromise choice of having only a small taste?

The reason we are so concerned that you not blow something out of proportion is that many times the urge for a single cookie will escalate to ten cookies as the fear and nervousness rises. It's like a poker game: when the stakes rise, so does the tension. In this case, the reverse process occurs. Tension is high, so you adjust the stakes accordingly: now it's ten cookies instead of one.

This tendency to see the scenerio as much worse than it is may lead you to abandon effort altogether if you don't control it. Don't ignore a week of success because you ate a single cookie or got off the bike five minutes earlier than you originally intended. Don't define yourself in terms of a small indulgence or a momentary fatigue. By seeing what effect this will have in the long run, you can ease your sense of failure and allow yourself to choose what you really want to do in the moment.

The ABCs
A: Examine your thoughts to identify your thinking styles.
B: Devise alternative ways to look at a situation. Ask yourself: What are the other ways of looking at this situation?

Make a list of alternatives and keep them handy.
What other ways can I act in this situation?
C: Consider the actual worst case scenerio.

Talking Your Way Out

Another way to overcome overwhelming intensity is to talk your way out. Let your Internal Director talk to the Sedentary Slob within you. First, however, you have to create an image of your Sedentary Slob, just as you created your wellness image.

Creating your Sedentary Slob

Have some fun with this exercise. Take a clipboard or a firm book and put a few pieces of paper on it. With a pencil in hand, find a comfortable chair. Be playful and powerful! This is not an exercise to take too seriously.

1. Take slow, deep diaphragmatic breaths. Do this for one or two minutes. To get in touch with an image of your Sedentary Slob, think of a recent episode when you felt captured by it. For example, if you were "too tired" to exercise on Tuesday, focus on how you felt. Allow whatever image comes to mind to develop. Use your imagination to fill in the details.

2. You can either write out a desription in words or draw it. How big is it? What is it wearing? Is it a human, an animal, or a plant? (We've heard it all.) What colour is it? Does it have a shape? Does it have body parts? (Some people have simply seen colours or objects.)

3. Repeat the exercise by imagining other times that you have been taken over by your Sedentary Slob role. Allow a few images to come to mind, then decide which has the most meaning for you.

4. Some people imagine themselves walking down a dark corridor and finding a door (perhaps a refrigerator door). They open the door and "see" their Sedentary Slob lying on the couch with a bag of chips, watching reruns on television.

Many images are simple. We have heard people describe green blobs, a huge mound of jello, a huge mouth with tiny arms and legs, or even a Venus fly trap. There is no definitive form that your Sedentary Slob should take, but it should be your own.

If you find this exercise making you either nervous or sad, that's fine. You're getting in touch with the feelings associated with being in the Sedentary Slob state. You can do a few things to ease the exercise if it gets too overwhelming:

1. Open your eyes and smile. Remember, playful and positive!
2. Choose to focus on a situation that will provoke less anxiety. Bring your wellness image to mind.
3. Smile as you do this exercise.

Write as many notes as you need while doing this exercise. If you get two or more images or your Sedentary Slob, then choose the one that you will enjoy bringing to mind. If you get an image that is too disturbing (a skeleton or some form that disgusts you), give the exercise up for now and try it again another time.

Talking Your Way Out

Once you have created your Sedentary Slob image, you can begin talking to it. Get comfortable. Visualize your Sedentary Slob walking out on a stage. Ask it questions – any questions you want. You might ask why it tries to control you or how it got started in the first place. Listen to what it says when it is leading you to make disease-promoting choices.

When we talk about listening to the Sedentary Slob, our patients often respond, "Listen to what?" The voice of your Sedentary Slob is in the thoughts that pop into your mind when you've asked it specific questions. By creating an image of your Sedentary Slob, you activate the part of your mind that has your unconscious blueprint for this part of you.

To see what we mean, try the following experiment. Ask yourself "What is your name?" An answer will pop immediately into your mind. In the same way, whatever thoughts come to mind when you imagine yourself talking to your Sedentary Slob are the answers you hear when you ask it questions. Some of its responses will seem silly or outrageous. Others, however, will give you a greater understanding of who you are.

After you have come to know your Sedentary Slob, you can begin to change your relationship with it by changing the conversation. The next time you encounter an overwhelming intensity moment, call up your Internal Director by using your diaphragmatic breathing. Approach your Sedentary Slob with one of the three methods described below. All three approaches attempt to modify your relationship with your Sedentary Slob. During these conversations, your vivid image of your Sedentary Slob may disappear and other thoughts may intrude. If this happens, just try to refocus and return to the dialogue.

There is no wrong time to perform these exercises, except when you are operating mechanical equipment, driving a car, or engaged in some other activity that requires your full attention. Whether you are alone or with a group of people, you can use these strategies in any challenging moment. Your success will depend on your willingness to develop an image of your Sedentary Slob, to give it an identity, and to visualize it.

The process of bringing your Sedentary Slob to mind will help you succeed in the long run. Initially, all you will experience with your eyes open is a vague feeling and image of your Sedentary Slob's outline. Eventually, the image will become more specific:

> I still see everything in front of me but there is this sense of my Sedentary Slob, that dough-boy from the commercial, in my mind. For a few fleeting seconds, I can make out the whiteness of his image or the buttons on his body, and then

the image is gone. I never actually see him, but I sense his presence. I get the same sense recalling his image as I do when remembering the layout of my bedroom or what a particular person looks like.

Approach Number 1: Greeting an Old Friend

In your overwhelming intensity state, you are often too anxious to succeed. When you visualize your Sedentary Slob, you are no longer playing that role. Instead, you separate yourself from it. Then you can change the intensity of the struggle by greeting your Sedentary Slob as an old friend. Try saying to your Sedentary Slob something like, "I was wondering where you'd been lately. I've actually missed your fat little face." Greet your Sedentary Slob (and the overwhelming intensity moment) with a confident smile on your face and an outstretched hand. Imagine shaking hands with it or giving it a hug, as you would with an old friend.

By greeting your Sedentary Slob, you are taking on the role of the Internal Director instead of accepting the Sedentary Slob role. Smiling is a powerful way to decrease the intensity of the struggle. Using funny responses in the moment of temptation will further increase your control of the situation.

This technique works well for some people. Laura, a 27-year-old homemaker, was finding she consistently ate too many sweets at family gatherings. We taught her how to recognize the moment and to step back from it. She started visualizing her Sedentary Slob sitting on whatever it was she wanted to eat. She'd say, in her mind, "It's good to see you! Where have you been? I've missed you. I know how much you'd like me to eat some of that chocolate mousse, but I am committed to more healthy choices now. Sorry."

Approach Number 2: Exaggerating the Outcome

Using this approach, you see your Sedentary Slob carrying out whatever action you fear, but you take it to an extreme. If doughnuts are your weakness, then imagine your Sedentary Slob gobbling 500 doughnuts. Watch it eat a truckload of chocolate bars. See your Sedentary Slob getting fatter, until buttons pop, clothes tear, and the poor beast finally explodes from overeating. Always carry the situation to the point of ridiculousness. Don't take the situation seriously; embellish it until you smile and giggle:

> Many times, at the beginning of a run, I really didn't feel up to the exercise. Tired or aggravated by something, I'd just want to stop. But then I'd imagine myself with a huge pot belly, shirt open at the waist, unsuccessfully trying to get up off the couch, trapped like a turtle on its back. Inevitably, this image made me smile and I would finish the run.

Approach Number 3: Make My Day

If you are feeling helpless or unsure whether you can make a wellness choice, you should probably greet your Sedentary Slob assertively. Pretend your're a gunslinger coming up against the notorious Sedentary Slob.

> Okay, fat boy. Just you try to get me. Make my day! I'm warning you, you'd better get me good. You used to be so good at getting me before, but I don't think you have it in you any more. I guess you're just too tired now. Maybe you're losing your touch.

Many of the people we have counselled have used this approach successfully. Barbara, a 23-year-old law student, used to go directly to the pizza shop after working in the library until midnight. No matter how often she reviewed her goals, she managed to avoid the pizza shop less than 50 percent of the time, even though she usually wasn't even hungry. She always felt that she was too weak to succeed. Then she began to challenge her Sedentary Slob as she walked from the library. She'd say, "Go ahead, give me your best shot. Just try to make me eat a slice of pizza." Moments later her anxiety would dissipate and she would be able to overcome her temptation.

Karen, a 31-year-old career counsellor and a mother of two, used to have trouble motivating herself to do her weight training. Regardless of how much she envisioned enjoying the benefits, she just could not get through the exercise. She then began to picture her Sedentary Slob leaning on the machine as she sat down. Imagining its extra weight spurred her into action. "No plump little body's going to stop me! Just watch!"

Be detailed and specific in your conversatons with your Sedentary Slob. If you find you can't remember the process at the times you need it, try writing your own versions of scenarios on index cards. Carry them with you so that you will be prepared when the moment arises.

Acting Your Way Out

Actors can communicate how their characters feel without even speaking. For many people, talking to themselves or visualizing is not as helpful as a change of posture, facial expression, and breathing. In an overwhelmed anxiety state, you are playing the role of the Sedentary Slob. Your Sedentary Slob has a specific way of acting that captures how you feel while you are playing that role. You probably breathe more quickly, slouch, have your eyes downcast, and frown. You may feel particularly self-conscious about your appearance. Break out of that Sedentary Slob role by electing to play a different part. If you stop acting like your Sedentary Slob, you will probably stop feeling like a Sedentary Slob.

By taking slow, deep diaphragmatic breaths, you can relax and step out of an overwhelming intensity state. Say "Cool air in" as you breathe in and "Warm air out" as you breathe out. Talk slowly so that it takes a second for you to say each word. While breathing, do exercises to improve your posture. Gently roll your shoulders back. Feel an imaginary rope pulling your head up as you straighten your posture. Hold your head up and smile, showing the world your sense of self-confidence.

Critical to acting your way out is the ability to feel and to move in a way that resonates with your wellness role. *You may find that visualizing your wellness image helps you establish a good attitude while you do these physical steps.*

The more you work with these particular exercises, the more powerful they will become. You will begin to develop a memory library of successes that will sustain you in future challenges. If you want to give this technique a chance to work, do it every day for 14 days. This is a new experience, and only with time will you really know if it works for you. Remember that it has taken years to develop the attitudes you have, so they can't possibly disappear overnight.

Exhibit 6-3
Switching Out of Overwhelming Intensity

Seeing Your Way Out

Advance Preparation:
Define your wellness image and visualize it daily.

In the Moment:
Step back into your Internal Director's role using diaphragmatic breathing.
Visualize your wellness image.

Thinking Your Way Out

Advance Preparation:
Become very familiar with the 10 thinking styles and the personal ways you use them.

In the Moment:
Step back and breate deeply.
Label your thinking style and assess how it affects the way you are thinking and acting.
Rewrite the script.

    a. Examine your thoughts to identify your thinking styles.
    b. Devise alternative ways to look at the situation.
    c. Consider the actual worst case senario.

Talking Your Way Out

Advance Preparation:
Create a detailed image of your Sedentary Slob.
As part of your visualization sessions, talk to your Sedentary Slob and get to know it.
If you think it will help, prepare scenarios on index cards so that you are ready for an unexpected crisis.

In the Moment:
Change the conversation by approaching your Sedentary Slob in one of three ways:
1. Greeting an Old Friend: Be friendly to your Sedentary Slob, treating it as an old friend.
2. Exaggerating the Outcome: Imagine your Sedentary Slob doing what what you want to do, then carry that to a ridiculous extreme.
3. Make My Day: Be assertive. Confront your Sedentary Slob as a gunslinger.

Acting Your Way Out

Advance Preparation:
Practice your diaphragmatic breathing and posturizing exercises. Develop your wellness image.

In the Moment:
Take several slow, deep breaths. To slow down your breathing, you can say "Cool air in" and "Warm air out" as you breathe.
Perform posture exercises – gently roll back your shoulders, stretch your body up without raising your arms, hold your head high, and smile.
Visualize your wellness image. See yourself step into your role. Feel the image spread through your body.

Starting Right Now . . .

1. Experiment with these techniques for switching out of overwhelming intensity: seeing your way out, thinking your way out, talking your way out, and acting your way out. Find the method or combination that works best for you. Practice so you will be ready to deal with a crisis when the moment arrives.

2. If you decide to talk your way out, write a description of the Sedentary Slob in the Wellness Planner (p. 316).

Switching Out of Insufficient Intensity

If you're watching television, eating a bowl of chips, enjoying a beer and a cigarette, and generally living the life of a couch potato, welcome to the comfort zone. In this state, feeling overwhelmed by wellness choices seems silly. Food is for enjoyment. Exercise is something to do when the channel changer is broken. You are experiencing insufficient intensity.

It's not only the couch potato or candy-club member who can slip into this state. Any time you automatically act out a health-related behavior without considering the health implications, you are probably in an insufficient intensity state. Anyone who has been involved in training over a long period of time could tell you that you can slip into this state if you let the pattern take over. If you find your commitment to exercise being eroded by monotony, you might need to try something different. Introduce some novelty or variety into your exercise pattern to help raise your intensity level.

Regardless of your wellness commitment, you can suddenly find yourself in an insufficient intensity state if you allow your routine to become boring or stale. Returning to the optimum health-promoting state can be accomplished by something as simple as trying some new recipes. What is crucial here is that you don't allow yourself to return to your former disease-promoting ways, but rather get back on track by adopting a new health-promoting step.

To get out of insufficient intensity, you need to increase your desire to achieve wellness, strengthen commitment, and abandon your comfort zone. The techniques we suggest integrate the knowledge you have learned from the rest of the Winning Weigh program and apply it in the moment of making a decision.

Every day, you have many opportunities to commit yourself to health. Each of these situations is not a great challenge in itself, but as a whole they determine who you will become, both physically and mentally. Here are just a few examples from a normal day:

- Will you have bacon and eggs or a high-fiber cereal for breakfast?
- Will you drink coffee all day or sip on mineral water flavored with lime?
- Will you choose salad or a hamburger for lunch?
- Will you snack on a crunchy apple or a chocolate bar?
- Will you walk five blocks to the store or take the car?
- Will you exercise at the end of the day or head straight for the couch?

The key is to recognize these moments as opportunities for change. Switch off automatic pilot mode. Stop and identify your choice. Step into your Internal Director's role and begin your diaphramatic breathing. Then use one of the three ways of switching from an insufficient intensity state: seeing your way out, thinking your way out, or acting your way out. Any of these three paths will increase your intensity to an optimal level.

Seeing Your Way Out

You can see your way out of insufficient intensity by visualizing the long-term risks and benefits of your choice at that moment. Move to your Internal Director's chair. Use the vivid and personal aspects of the risk to break through all of your attempts to deny the potential damage of your decisions. Faced with a decision about whether to eat an apple or chocolate cake, try a visualization like the one below.

Health Visualization
See your cholesterol dragged through your intestinal tract by the cholesterol cruncher fiber in the apple. Next, watch your coronary arteries clearing and widening. Envision the apple's beta-carotene trapping and gobbling up free radicals from the surface lining of your lungs, stomach, and bladder. See a thinner, shapelier you emerge as you reduce your body fat. Imagine how energetic and vibrant you are.

Disease Visualization

Imagine your coronary arteries filling up with tiny pieces of cholesterol. See your heart working harder to pump enough blood to your cells. Feel pains in your chest and imagine yourself lying in a hospital bed with tubes coming from your arms and nose. Really see what happens as the chocolate cake blocks your arteries.

Seeing your way out requires that you be familiar with much of the information that you learned in Step 2: Focusing on the Benefits. In the two visualizations above, you needed to know the effects of high-fat foods on your coronary arteries to create the image. We cannot take you through every possible food or activity, listing the potential health-promoting or disease-promoting images. To succeed in achieving your long-term goals, you'll need to transform the information you learned in Step 2 into an image like the one in the above example.

By imagining the long-term effects of your choices vividly, you intimately link the effect with you. The immediate, short-term gratification is no longer standing alone; it is overbalanced by the effects of your choices on your body.Once you have really viewed the alternatives, you are prepared to make a more committed choice for healthy action.

Thinking Your Way Out

Many people find it more natural to think than to visualize. You can use your knowledge of nutrition to do a risk/benefit analysis, incorporating nutritional facts into usable personal knowledge. Break your analysis down into immediate, short-term, and long-term risks and benefits. We are likely to choose food on the basis of taste. By focusing on the ***long-term*** benefits and risks, you will view the choice entirely differently – you bring the impact of your day-to-day decisions into perspective. No one dies after having one slice of bread mounded with butter. However, the day-to-day choices add up to your individual wellness or disease. Remember that 50 percent of the population dies of heart disease and 40 percent of cancer deaths are diet-related.

Let's say you are about to eat chocolate cake without really thinking about it. You realize this is a moment of insufficient intensity. After identifying your choices, you assess the risks and benefits, thus shifting your viewpoint from a comfort zone to a conscious decision between disease-promoting or health-promoting behavior. This action eliminates the disconnection between what you know and what you do. Confront your decision in the moment. You can still choose not to act on your knowledge. Remember in the end to accept whichever choice you make. Exhibit 6–4 provides an example of a risk/benefit analysis for eating an apple versus eating chocolate cake.

Acting Your Way Out

An actor can take on a role even if he or she has not fully adopted the part yet. To take on your wellness part, you simply have to step into your wellness image. This image will give you some perspective on why you are bothering with wellness at all.

Let's say it is Sunday morning and you usually go for a run, but today you think you are just not interested. You recognize an insufficient intensity moment, so you step into your wellness image, drawing on its energy. You can be the person you want to be. Step into the runner's role. Become the runner in your mind's eye. By focusing energy and effort, you can draw from the enthusiasm and commitment that helped you create the image in the first place. See your wellness image and feel it spread through your body. Head up, shoulders back, smile in place, gently take on the physical feeling of your wellness image. Once you recapture the sense of how exciting your wellness image is, you will probably find the energy to go for that run.

Your Wellness Journey

How should you feel on the Winning Weigh program? Is it OK to feel the urge to eat an old disease-promoting favorite? Will your urges for chocolate disappear if you're on the program for months? To better understand how it feels during the period of change, imagine yourself watching two plays being acted out. You have the lead role in both plays. The stage on the left stars you in either your insufficient or your overwhelming intensity script. That is your old part. The stage on the right features you in your new script, called "My Wellness Story."

All along, long before you started reading this book, you have made health- and disease-promoting choices, acting out one of the two scenes. By following the seven steps of **The Winning Weigh,** you are building a stage and developing the dialogue to play out your wellness script as your principal role. In time, the disease-promoting script will begin to fade and be less pronounced, but in the right setting your mood or other people will activate the old story line, which will be as powerful as ever. You need to accept this fact and prepare for it.

Even after six months of making health-promoting choices in a consistent manner, you will still hear the dialogue of your blissful binge scene pass through your head. Many get concerned with this surge of the past but it is simply an indicator that the old script is still present and you just have to recognize its presence. So when you find yourself struggling with a feeling that the program doesn't work or you are too tired to perform the Winning Weigh in-the-moment exercises, you need to remember that you are moving to the left stage and are acting out one more episode of your overwhelming-intensity script starring you as your Sedentary Slob. By expecting both lifestyle scripts to be present, you will better understand the challenge of living in the moment.

Put simply, you are always faced with choices. By watching carefully you can recognize which of the two scripts you are acting out in a given moment. By seeing the repetitive quality of the two scripts you tend to play, you are taking the first step back. With that perspective you should see that you can change in this very moment.

For each of the following techniques, step back into your Internal Director's role using diaphramatic breathing.

Seeing Your Way Out

In the Moment:
- Visualize either the disease-promoting or health-promoting effects of your alternative courses of action. Make the images as vivid as possible.

Thinking Your Way Out

In the Moment:
- Identify the choices you have in that moment.
- Assess the risks and benefits, thus shifting your viewpoint from the comfort zone to a conscious decision between disease-promoting and health-promoting behavior.

Acting Your Way Out

In the Moment:
- Step into your wellness image. Imagine putting on the image like a piece of clothing. Become the enthusiastic, committed person that you have envisioned.

The Method in Five Scenes

By reviewing five short scenes, we will show you the in-the-moment techniques in action. You can see how two scripts unfold at once.

Scene One

BJ is a 35-year-old businessman who came to see us 20 pounds overweight and living the salad-ice cream diet. That's when the foods you eat are either extremely health-promoting or very much in the disease-promoting category. We take you now to an early point in his Winning Weigh program.

"I find myself in the kitchen late at night saying 'I really feel like a piece of cake or a couple pieces of bread with butter.' Despite having read over my goals in the morning, I am suddenly anxiously wanting bread. Finding myself compelled to eat, I begin to butter a piece of fresh rye bread and think about defrosting a bagel. I shut the refrigerator door and I see my sign that reads 'I am committed to wellness each and everyday.'"

Still maintaining a sense of humor, BJ adds "thank goodness it's nighttime."

Realizing that he is about to act out a scene of his insufficient intensity, he becomes anxious and frightened that he'll just never change. He has shifted into an overwhelming intensity state. One thing he has learned and enjoys is stepping into his Internal Director role, and he quickly takes three deep breaths and steps back. He can now clearly see the two opportunities. It is as if the curtain comes up on the wellness stage.

Reviewing his thoughts he hears:
"I'll just eat the bread and butter, but starting tommorow . . . I am such a loser, I'll never be able to do this." And he angrily grabs the plate and begins to eat.

Quickly, he labels the first thought as procrastination and the second as blaming himself, realizing that "by blaming myself for being so weak, I was already remorseful for what I hadn't yet done. This was a step away from giving myself permission."

He goes back to watching television, leaving the buttered bread unfinished. Within a minute he feels the mild nervous feeling come back and a tightness in his throat that accompanied his fear that he would still act in keeping with his Sedentary Slob role. Going to his deep breathing, he quickly calms himself. He remembers that he has a peach in the fridge. Tossing the bread in the garbage, he commits himself to eating the peach instead. Walking quickly, a smile on his face and his head held high, BJ feels his intensity level shifting with each step he takes. As he takes out the fruit, he quickly reviews its value for fiber and essential vitamins, including antioxidants. He truly enjoys the fruit. (He described to us how sweet it was and how his surprise at how good it tasted. Many people on the Winning Weigh program are surprised to discover how wonderful fruit tastes.)

BJ has been quite successful since beginning the program five years ago. He lost and has kept off his 20 excess pounds, he enjoys working out four times a week, and he has found meditation to be a valued addition to his busy life. By making one in-the-moment decision after another, BJ was able to develop a strong, effective wellness role.

Scene Two

Emily, a busy advertising executive who rarely gets a chance to eat when she'd like to, carried ten extra pounds and was constantly tired, anxious, and suffering from a general feeling of "wanting to get out of my skin." She came to see us about this stress. She quickly adopted the eating portion of the Winning Weigh program, but still felt as anxious. We advised her to begin doing regular exercise, for both her mental and physical well- being.

She had trouble motivating herself to work out. After a long day, She wanted to just go home and relax. On the day that we join her, she is just leaving her office. She is still unsure where she is going – home or to the fitness club. Grabbing her briefcase and gym bag, she heads for the elevator. On the elevator, heading down, she struggles with the two options, until she says to herself "Fine, I need to go to my breathing." Breathing slowly, she brings her wellness image to mind. In detail she sees her realistic image: her hair tied up; a baggy t-shirt with a one-piece workout suit underneath; socks and white running shoes; moving up and down on the stairmaster. She enjoys that image, smiles, and uses the image to guide her toward the gym.

She walks to the gym quickly, at almost double her usual pace. Swinging her arms, she feels her intensity level shifting with every step she takes. Simple as this method seems, she is regularly exercising three times a week. By getting to the gym often enough, she has become hooked on the idea of working out. The image can often be a transitional motivator until the pleasure of just working out takes over.

Scene Three

Fifty pounds overweight and a former member of ten weight-loss self-help groups, Bob entered the first session saying "You can't help me, but my family doctor told me to come see you." Off-and-on diabetic, working ten-hour days, and out of shape, he was a physical mess. He had all the warning signs of heart disease. He was also one of the angriest people we had ever met.

We decided to let him set his own involvement level. He had only one passion besides his children — fishing around his cottage. He looked forward to retiring and spending his time there three seasons a year. I'll never forget the look on his face when we said to him, "The only thing you'll have to do with fishing when you are 65 is as bait." This image of him as dead by then was not taken well. He left, letting us know that he would not be back.

Three months later, he returned saying "I'm ready to change." As it turned out, one of his closest friends had dropped dead of a heart attack. This was the fear incentive that he needed to get moving in changing his life. He had come back to us because, as he put it, "You were blunt and to the point."

Bob's attitude was "I can do what I want, so don't tell me what to do." We tried to help him change by focusing on the benefits he could expect from eating well and taking care of himself. We tapped into his hopes, dreams, and expectations.

We identified many individual examples of his pleasures and dreams and helped him relate them to his overall health. Did we scare him? Let's just say we didn't hold back on telling him of the complications of diabetes, stress, and living an obese life. The risks did not match up favorably against his long-term goals. He wanted to chase after his grandchildren (he turned out to be quite sentimental) and to be able to walk in the woods with his wife in his sixties.

He worked well with analytic thinking, so we taught him to use the risk and benefits chart (see Exhibit 6-4, p. 269). In each situation, he would evaluate his options in terms of immediate. short-term, and long-term benefits. Bacon and eggs for breakfast began to seem useless, and his afternoon chocolate bar was just too fattening, not to mention what it did to his sugars level. The risk of losing a leg or part of a foot because of gangrene brought on by diabetes activated his fears of being dependent and passive. By enhancing this thought into a visual image of him in a wheelchair looking at the fishing dock from the cottage window, he developed a technique for keeping himself on track.

We encouraged him to join a weight-reduction clinic, and he faithfully attended their meetings as well as completing our eight-week program. Working with his family doctor, we developed a walking program, and he went to a health spa to develop a healthy attitude toward cooking and being associated with wellness.

One year later, he had lost 45 pounds. He rode the exercise bike six days a week and was on the vegetarian version of the two-staple system. Still not a friendly person, he found it most helpful to use images of him being passive and weak because of some disease to help avoid his disease-promoting actions. Many times it is the recognition of what we are afraid will happen to us, in this case being dependent, that drives us to get on track.

Scene Four

MR was a couch potato until he started jogging regularly. On many occasions, he had watched friends and family enjoy long-distance running, but he had always "been amazed that they could do it." It was this admiration for their special ability that kept him from trying it. He never thought of himself as an athlete, so he assumed such activities were beyond him. Finding himself 15 pounds overweight and very jealous of a close friend who was a runner, he came to see us saying "I'd like to start running." This is always a strange request, considering that the obvious response, if there are no physical limitating factors, is "All right, start."

Going beyond this initial reaction, we discovered an all-or-nothing attitude to running. He believed if he couldn't run as far as his friends, there was no point in trying. Of course, his friends had been running for five years, but he didn't seem to see this as an important consideration.

We put him on a schedule that increased his distance by a half mile every four weeks, and he began to run. For about two months, he'd run four times one week and none the next. The next step was to put a calendar on his refrigerator (the best use for a refrigerator) and give him gold stars to stick on the day he ran. This elementary reward system got him running four times a week consistently. The rest of his health and wellness program came into focus without effort.

Exhibit 6–4
Risk/Benefits Analysis

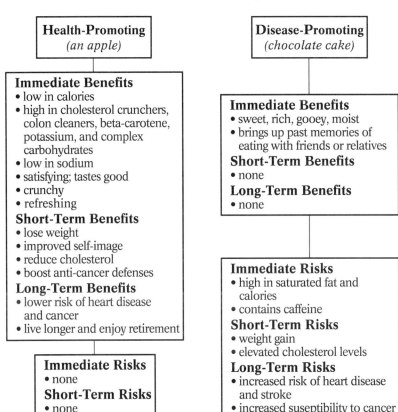

Last year MR ran his second marathon. This year he hopes to run a third and even a fourth. His friends have all stopped running, but he has continued. Injury free, endurance bound, he has proven to be a real competitor, but first he had to get beyond the idea that running is "for my really fit friends. No way I'd run for two hours every weekend day."

People can do a lot more than they imagine.

Scene Five

JP worked out three times a week on the stationary bicycle, followed a regular weight-training program, and enjoyed competitive games of hockey and baseball. He enjoyed eating fruits and vegetables but found it difficult to lower his fat intake because of his love for pizza, muffins, and other recreational foods. He realized he needed to cut back on the amount of fat in his diet, as there was a family history of hypertension, high cholesterol, and heart disease, but he always seemed to be starting tomorrow.

His relaxed easy-going nature made him feel that he was somehow protected from these dangers. However, in a routine exam for insurance purposes, JP discovered that his cholesterol was in the "high normal" range. This meant that he was at a 50 percent greater risk of heart disease than the average North American, not the kind of odds you'd like to take to Las Vegas. Considerably less casual about his health, he began to focus on switching his ways. But dinner parties, late-night snacks with the boys after a game, and the traditional slice of pizza for lunch were proving to be tougher to give up than he'd realized.

JP was caught in what we call the Health Club comfort zone. He worked out enough to have the cosmetic and superficial signs of being fit – thin, shapely, and firm – but underneath there was a real potential for serious health problems. To help motivate him out his comfort zone, we used the health-promotion and disease-promotion visualization technique (described on pages 260-261). People in the Health Club comfort zone generally respond well to this technique. JP managed to lower his daily fat intake to a safer 15-20 percent and consequently his cholesterol count also dropped. In addition, he lost the five extra pounds he had carried as love handles.

Starting Right Now . . .

Experiment with these techniques for switching out of an insufficient intensity moment: seeing your way out, thinking your way out, and acting your way out. Find the combination that works best for you.

Practice so you are ready to deal with a moment when you should abandon your comfort zone. Keep a record of your personal in-the-moment techniques using the diary on page 325. See the sample on page 323.

Summary For Step 6

1. Every day you face an abundance of opportunities to apply the Winning Weigh principles.

2. Every decision is influenced by an overwhelming, optimum, or insufficient intensity level. By following our in-the-moment techniques, you can switch out of your automatic way of being, assess your intensity, and then step into a more appropriate mindset for achieving your goal.

3. By combining commitment with action you will empower your wellness role.

4. Review the different strategies for seeing, thinking, and acting your way out of the overwhelming and insufficient intensity levels. Commit yourself to applying the different options until you discover the combination of steps that works for you.

5. Remember: Be Playful! Be Powerful!

LOOKING AHEAD . . .

In Step 6, we concentrated all of the first five steps into the moment of making a health-promoting decision. In Step 7, we will outline the necessary daily commitments to help build your health-promoting attitude.

Step 7 provides the mental training that allows you to embrace your wellness choices in the moment. This final step keeps you on track by building a rational middle-of-the-road approach to your health. It will help you avoid slipping into the blissful binge or the perfect forever fantasy.

STEP 7: BECOMING THE GOAL TODAY

Staying on Track

Throughout this book, we have tried to show you how to evaluate your present dietary and exercise habits. We have also encouraged you to incorporate some basic wellness strategies into your life. Whether you have been on the wrong track for your whole life or have just slipped a bit lately, we hope *The Winning Weigh* has motivated you to take better care of your body. At the same time, you should develop an attitude of compassionate commitment. You will not stop being tempted by the foods you are in the habit of eating, so don't be too hard on yourself if you slip once in a while. It takes time before the new patterns will feel like your natural approach to life.

If exercise, even a simple walking program, doesn't feel comfortable to you in the beginning, stick with it anyway. Forgive yourself little slips, and concentrate on the long haul. This is lifetime stuff. In time, you will discover what a healthy, energizing, mood-enhancing addiction it can be.

You developed your goals in Step 4 of this program. By now, you should have started to feel emotionally connected to the positive outcomes that the Winning Weigh program will bring to your life. Now you need a strategy to keep yourself on track until you are consistently and automatically living your new existence and it feels completely natural to you.

As you probably realize from other experiences, one of the toughest things in life is remaining motivated today about the goals we set for ourselves yesterday. There is a trite but true saying that addresses this problem: "Success is 10 percent inspiration and 90 percent perspiration." If you really want to get to your goal, you need to work to stay on course.

There is a magical feeling that accompanies setting out to accomplish a big goal in your life. A new plan for success is always something to get excited about. Yet how many times have you set off enthusiastically to accomplish a goal only to discover that your zest for achievement insidiously slipping away soon after? It's easy to understand how this can happen. You probably deal with many pressures, demands, and choices every day. Because you are pulled in so many directions at once – careers, family, social activities – finding the time and energy to maintain the commitment to a new goal can be difficult.

Certainly this is true for wellness goals. Identifying what you want, committing it to paper, and planning how to go after it are exciting activities. Staying on track every day requires continual commitment and focus. Like any goal that involves new skills, reaching your wellness goals requires a daily effort until the changes in your lifestyle become a natural part of your life, requiring little thought. Daily activities accumulate over the years until they become habits.

Expect your old destructive habits to put up a strong fight. You will be tempted to fall back into your old comfort zone at the first sign of stress or fatigue. Watching television requires less motivation than walking or jogging. The grocery stores are filled with your favorite high-fat foods, all temptingly displayed. There is a fast-food restaurant or doughnut shop at almost every intersection in North America. Your Sedentary Slob and Self-Righteous Snob activators can steer you off course if you're not prepared. To resist these temptations, you need a strategy for staying on track until the principles of the Winning Weigh program become your accustomed pattern of behavior. A good image to hold in mind is that you are alone at sea in a sailboat heading toward your personal paradise. The winds may change from day to day, but they can only blow you off course if you fail to adjust the position of your sail regularly.

You may have tried to change your eating or exercise habits before, only to give up after a couple of days, weeks, or months. Initial enthusiasm doesn't guarantee that you will carry on with your good intentions after the fire has gone out. To break out of your comfort zone, you need a plan for staying on track every day so you don't lose ground as time goes by. Your formula for daily achievement must be in line with your long-range goals. Each day becomes one step in your journey.

We recommend you do three things every day and three things every week to strengthen your ability to make positive health-promoting decisions in the moment.

The Three Daily Steps

The following three actions are the most powerful ammunition we can provide to help you make in-the-moment health-promoting decisions all day long: familiarize, visualize, diarize. These procedures are critical if you want to stay on track and prevent your enthusiasm from being lost in the daily shuffle of life.

1. Familiarize: Review your goals and read your Wellness Planner each morning to set the direction of your sail.
The beginning of each new day is a critical time. Use that time to turn to the Wellness Planner and review your plan for accomplishing your goals. This simple action will prepare you for the tasks ahead of you that day. It will remind you of the importance of meeting your wellness intentions. It's simple, but it really does work. Failing to read your planner and review your goals will allow those resolutions you have made to fade slowly away. Your wellness plans will lose their place on your priority list if you don't remind yourself how important they are every day.

Making changes and new choices in your life requires a bit of extra effort in the beginning. Keep yourself focused on your goals until these changes became a natural extension of your life – until you have internalized them.

Reviewing your goals each day is the way to set the direction of your sail so that no matter how turbulent the winds of life may blow, you stay on your long-term course with the things that are important to you. Don't skip this part of the process: it only takes two or three minutes each day, but it can make the difference between succeeding with your wellness goals or losing ground until you're back to old destructive habits.

2. Visualize: Take five to ten minutes to visualize your wellness image and perform your breathing relaxation techniques.
The most powerful way to become connected to your wellness goals is through the use of the visualization technique you learned in Step 5.

With the help of breathing exercises, it will get you into a relaxed state of mind and enable you to focus on your wellness image and the benefits that are part of a health-promoting lifestyle. You will find this technique reduces stress and prepares you to deal with the challenges of the day ahead.

3. Diarize: Fill out the Daily Food, Fiber, and Activity Journal at the end of each day, as a means of monitoring your progress.
To ensure that you are doing your best to follow your nutritional and exercise program, you need to keep a record of your performance, at least until you are following the program automatically and it is no longer a struggle to stay on track. Look at the Food, Fiber, and Activity Journal on pages 323-324. At the end of each day, you should use that format to record the foods you've eaten, indicating the low-fat flesh and dairy protein meals and the complex-carbohydrate-only meal. Remember that you are aiming for the following:

one low-fat dairy protein meal
one low-fat flesh protein meal
one carbohydrate-only meal
8 to 15 fiber points
a maximum of two servings of olive or peanut oil
6 to 8 glasses of water
at least two foods containing anti-cancer protective nutrients.

Besides tracking your eating patterns, you can review your Food, Fiber, and Activity Journal to see whether you are slipping back into eating foods from the recreational or hazardous categories. You will find that the mere task of picking up a pen and reporting to yourself on paper will often stop your from slipping into bad habits. The Food, Fiber, and Activity Journal will work as a powerful deterrent to eating foods that will drive you off track. It will also strengthen your commitment to your exercise program. At the end of each week, you can really see what pattern of conduct is emerging.

From our experience and from the research of other authorities, this self-monitoring is one of the most effective ways to keep to the path you have set for yourself. People who keep daily food and activity records perform much better in the long term than people who don't keep any records.

The Evolution Process

As you follow these three techniques for staying on track, your daily performance will improve. You may struggle a little at the beginning, but time, experience, and repetition will suddenly produce a breakthrough for you. At some point in the first three months, you'll begin to experience the benefits of your efforts. You will lose some fat and some weight. Your clothes will start to fit better. You will have more energy. You'll feel more fit and you'll look healthier. Even your taste buds will undergo a transformation as you begin to prefer fish over spare ribs, tomato sauce over cream sauce, and fruit over chocolate bars. The day will come when not exercising will feel unnatural and a new pattern of eating is an ingrained part of your life.

The Three Weekly Steps

In addition to the three daily strategies for staying on track, there are three things you should do on a weekly basis that will help to ensure your success.

1. Find the time to exercise by planning your workout time in advance.

One of the most common stumbling blocks for people trying to follow the Winning Weigh program is that they don't find time for exercise. The only way to overcome this problem is to plan your exercise time in advance. At the start of each week, take a look at all the things you are planning to do for the next seven days. Look at work commitments, family commitments, social functions, hair cuts, doctor's appointments, and anything else you know of. Get a clear picture in advance of how your week is shaping up. Then decide on which days and at what times you plan to exercise. Remember, you must exercise at least three times per week, spaced out as evenly as possible.

If you fail to plan for exercise time, you probably just won't get around to it. When you write it down in your weekly planner, you're making a commitment to yourself to follow through. Inevitably, you will find yourself juggling some plans in the middle of the week, but you know that exercise is important to your health, so be sure you always include time for it.

If you don't have the time to exercise, that probably just means that you haven't made it a high enough priority. Exercise is a fundamental requirement of maintaining a healthy body. You cannot change that truth because you don't like it or you're having trouble fitting it into a busy schedule.

Our experience has shown us that people who are willing to get up a little earlier in the morning to do their workout tend to have the best long-term compliance overall. If you leave your exercise until later in the day, something else may come up unexpectedly and you'll end up taking care of what seems urgent in the moment rather than what is is essential in the long term.

However, not everyone is a morning person, so you must go with your own body rhythm. The two authors of this book take different approaches. Barry Simon likes to get up early and run five to ten miles or do an aerobic workout on a cross-country ski machine for an hour. Jim Meschino prefers to do his aerobic workout in the evening as a means of winding down and reducing the stress of the day.

After a while, you'll find your workout time so rejuvenating that you won't need us to insist on its importance any more. In fact, you'll find that you develop a healthy addiction to it and if you go without exercise, you'll feel sluggish and out of sorts. And then you'll be like us – unable to understand people who say they can't find the time to exercise. Plan the time and get on with it. Make the time to exercise at least three times per week.

2. Make up a weekly Winning Weigh shopping list.
It's important to restock your kitchen with Winning Weigh foods

every week. To ensure that you surround yourself with healthy foods, make a shopping list. Don't buy junk food that might tempt you during a weak moment.

And along the same lines, stop baking for the people you love! Many people enjoy baking all kinds of dessert treats for their family and friends. We hate to disappoint you, but baking is no longer an acceptable way of showing your love for the people you care about. Feeding them high-fat and sugar-sweetened pies, cakes, and cookies promotes the development of heart disease, diabetes, and other degenerative diseases – hardly a considerate gift. We know this isn't your intention, but that's exactly what you're doing. Express your love by preparing healthy alternatives to disease-promoting foods such as fruit salads and occasional sherbets.

3. Fill Out a Weekly Body Shape Summary.
If part of your motivation for trying the Winning Weigh program is that you are trying to change your weight or figure, then it is important to measure your weekly progress. The Weekly Body Shape Summary is an excellent yardstick for measuring and reviewing how your body shape is changing. Too often, our patients become hung up on weighing themselves over and over again. The truth is, the scale is the least important tool for assessing wellness changes. You can easily lose excess body fat and look more slender on the Winning Weigh program yet increase your weight because of the increased storage of carbohydrates in your liver and skeletal muscles, especially at the beginning of the program. It is important to measure these changes in your body shape so that you realize a body transformation is under way. Recording these measurements will help reinforce your success and strengthen your determination to keep going. We have supplied you with two Weekly Body Shape Summaries on pages 326 and 327. Make some copies of this form, and insert one for each week in your Daily Food, Fiber, and Activity Journal.

Bring in the Reinforcements

As well as the three weekly and three daily strategies for staying on track, we have additional techniques you can use to keep your commitment alive. Try some of the approaches listed in the following pages to reinforce your determination.

1. Health Magazines
If you are going to get into the wellness lifestyle, you will want to learn more about recent scientific research relating to health. We have invariably found that people who continue to educate themselves remain more connected to a way of living that promotes wellness. As doctors interested in prolonging the quality of our patients' lives, we continually read through the latest research material at a highly technical level. We are aware of how much reading these papers every month reinforces our own commitment to wellness principles in our day-to-day lives. However, several excellent health magazines are available that translate academic findings into everyday language for the layperson. We especially recommend the following. As a rule, the articles are well-written, easy to understand, and accurate.

Longevity   *Men's Health*
In-Health   *Health*
Shape   *Runner's World*

You don't have to subscribe to all of them. Go to a magazine stand and flip through the pages. Find one or two that appeal to you and subscribe. You'll be amazed how their arrival at your home every month will affect your wellness commitment. They'll help the Winning Weigh principles continue to evolve to be a natural part of your life. Reading the positive, up-to-date information will be a potent and powerful influence for staying on track from month to month.

2. Audio and Video Tapes
The consumer market is flooded with audio and video tapes aimed at

the health, nutrition, and fitness markets. Just like health magazines, they can give you the reinforcement you need to stay on track. If you don't want to join a fitness club, an aerobic fitness video may be a good way to work out. Once again, the more you learn about wellness, the better your chances are for succeeding in the long term. And in health, the long term is what matters.

3. Pictures

You know the old cliché "a picture's worth a thousand words." Help yourself stay on track with your wellness goals by posting up a picture of a trim, fit person cut out from a magazine. Put it where you will see it at least twice a day. Remember, your goals have to be believable, so choose a picture that shows a body and activity within your reach. When you see this picture every day on your bedroom wall, on your mirror, on your desk, over the sink, or on the refrigerator door, it will help you visualize your goal.

Instead of someone from a magazine, you could use a photo of yourself when you were at your peak of physical fitness. This photo might be more effective than a picture of someone else, because it provides the physical evidence that you can succeed.

4. Quotes

Quotations and sayings can have the same effect as pictures. If it is meaningful to you, a positive quotation can inspire you to greater effort. It can help you create a positive, productive, powerful, and playful feeling that will improve your performance. Find positive quotes and put them where you will see them each day. Some of our favorites include

> If it is to be, it's up to me.

> Whoever wants to reach a distant goal must take many small steps. (Helmut Schmidt)

> We all count in this life – whether negatively or positively. It's each individual's own choice.

You can't change the world, but you can change yourself.

I never knew a man worth his salt who, in the long run, deep down in his heart, did not appreciate the grind and discipline necessary to become a champion. (Vince Lombardi)

5. Getting Enough Rest
Breaking out of your present comfort zone requires some energy at first. The extra energy required may leave you feeling tired in the early stages. When you feel tired, you'll lose your initial enthusiasm and your natural tendency will be to fall back into your old way. You should fight that tired feeling by either going to bed half an hour earlier than usual every night or catching a power nap sometime during the day. You'll be amazed at how much better you'll feel and how much easier it will be to stay on track with your wellness goals.

6. Positive People
Every year since the early 1970s, thousands of people join the wellness movement. These positive, high-energy people of all ages can be a tremendous source of inspiration if you get close enough for the effects to rub off. You do not need to copy their exact lifestyle or fitness routine, but allow their positive attitudes to recharge your mental battery.

Joining a fitness club can also put you in contact with men and women of all ages who are involved in a wellness lifestyle. Make sure the club is conveniently located so you can just drop in regularly. If it is too far out of your way, you won't use it regularly. Take an aerobics class, an aqua-fitness class, or a seniors' fitness class. Get to know other people who are tuned into the wellness philosophy. Surround yourself with the people who can help you succeed.

Remember that attitudes are contagious. Don't let a few negative people pull you off the road to a better life. Don't be influenced by self-defeating attitudes. Ultimately, you know what is in your best interest. Not everyone shares the same philosophy on life. Some people are content to smoke two packs of cigarettes a day, eat junk food, and pay no heed to preventive health. If that's the way they think, so be it. But why let them divert you from your goals? Those people who boldly and fearlessly proclaim that they are here for a good time may change their minds after sustaining their first heart attack. Only you can know what you really want for yourself.

7. The Winning Weigh
One of the best ways of staying on track is to read ***The Winning Weigh*** three or four times from cover to cover. Each time you read ***The Winning Weigh***, new information will jump off the page and new ideas will be triggered in your mind. While rereading the book, focus on how to fit the strategies into your day-to-day life.

Starting Right Now . . .

Do the following every day:
1. Review your goals and read your Wellness Planner each morning.
2. Take 15 to 20 minutes each day to visualize your wellness image and perform your breathing relaxation techniques. The morning is the best time.
3. Fill out the Daily Food, Fiber, and Activity Journal at the end of each day as a means of self-monitoring.

Do the following every week:
1. Find the time to exercise by planning your workout time in advance.
2. Make up a weekly Winning Weigh shopping list.
3. Fill out a Weekly Body Shape Summary.

Use these reinforcements to help keep yourself on track:
1. Health magazines.
2. Audio and video tapes.
3. Pictures.
4. Quotes.
5. Getting enough rest.
6. Positive people.
7. The Winning Weigh.

The Wellness Shift

Wellness is the active pursuit of mental, physical, and spiritual health every day. It is active because you not only prevent disease, but you improve your health through your conscious choices, guiding your own success. By regarding wellness as a lifetime of in-the-moment choices, you have an almost infinite number of opportunities to promote your health. By joining us in this active approach, you will begin to pursue wellness in a spirit of celebration instead of desperation – desperation to be thinner, faster, better looking, richer, or any of the other dreams that our society dangles before us as proofs of success. We encourage you to adopt your own goals rather than dreaming second-hand dreams.

There is a story told of a priest who was supervising the construction of the magnificent Notre Dame cathedral. During the building of the foundation, the priest walked up to a worker and asked him what he was doing. "I'm digging a ditch," the man replied. "What does it look like I'm doing?" Walking further, the priest asked a second ditch digger the same question. The second man exclaimed, "I'm building a cathedral!"

You may have started this program with an "I'm digging a ditch" attitude. You'll wonder how the small tasks we have laid out in the Winning Weigh fit together. You'll question the need to use in-the-moment techniques, and you'll wonder why you need to bother with the staying-on-track steps. Yet these small tasks, combined together, will help you recapture your lost love affair with your body and your health.

Turn your eyes inward and see the strengths you already have, the things you can do, the health you are starting with. Then you will begin your wellness journey from the only place you ever could begin – where you are right now. We have been committed in **The Winning Weigh** to teaching you basic nutritional information, to helping you set goals, to making you see beyond your old obstacles, to providing tools that you can use to stay on track for a lifetime.

A Tao teaching says, "A thousand-mile journey begins with one single step." We have taken you a few miles and given you the map for the next hundred, but it is up to you to search out other wisdom along the way. You must continue to modify your beliefs based on your experience and knowledge.

By combining commitment with health-promoting choices, you will begin to change. You were born with a great deal of potential to live a healthy life, yet you may have slowly lost this potential by making disease-promoting decisions. By the time you have reached this point in your reading, you have probably begun to change. Your daily actions are a reflection of your new wellness commitments.

So take it all slowly . . . one step at a time. If you walked a mile yesterday, then commit yourself to walking a little farther today. This ongoing process of change will dramatically increase your enthusiasm for wellness. But go slowly, respecting the quality that must accompany commitment if you are to have long-term success – compassion. Show compassion to your present health, to your genetic weaknesses, and to your own potential. By focusing on both compassion and commitment, you will find yourself a gradual but progressive health journey.

Remind yourself that you are not digging a ditch — you are building a cathedral. This is a slow but methodical process. There is a tale of a man who was frantically running along the street in New York City looking for the famous Carnegie Hall. He ran up to an elderly woman and asked her, "How do I get to Carnegie Hall?" The woman looked him up and down and said, "Practice, young man, practice." In order to succeed with the Winning Weigh techniques, you will need to practice each step of the exercises again and again.

You generate a great deal of power by practicing. Seeing yourself improve gives you a boost of what is called ***accomplishment feedback.*** Perform a committed action once and you'll want to try it again. Do it a hundred times and you'll begin to see yourself differently. Double that and other people will begin to see you differently. This principle applies to nearly everything in life. It is the feedback from a changing view of yourself that leads to accomplishment.

Practice is a critical ingredient in this process. You don't play a great symphony without practicing the scales. We've told you over and over that we don't expect you to succeed without some setbacks, but the principle of incremental improvement will be working for you. Your continued efforts will ultimately lead to a more positive and automatic pattern of behaving and acting. Some of the in-the-moment exercises or staying-on-track steps might seem unnecessary. However, when you slip back to your low-energy and vulnerable state, this solid foundation of practice will make it much easier to bounce back to an optimistic wellness frame of mind. Practice will lead your unconscious to adopt the Winning Weigh principles.

Despite all of your efforts to succeed on the Winning Weigh program, you will continue to experience the thoughts and beliefs of your Sedentary Slob. Don't worry about this tendency. The secret of success is your ability to simply step back onto the health-promoting track.

We would like to remind you of the definition of luck – opportunity meeting preparation. The Winning Weigh is your beginner's course in being prepared while you confront the daily opportunities to change your physical health and your unconscious views. Each moment that you are alive is truly an opportunity to experiment, to watch and be amazed by life.

Creating physical, mental, and spiritual health is a ongoing process. You can fool yourself into believing you can take breaks, but in fact it is all one long, continuous journey. It is impossible to start tomorrow or next week. Each moment is joined with the past moment. To try to take a break from your health is like saying, "I'm tired of breathing. I'll start again tomorrow."

As you read the last paragraph of this book, begin to think of the resources, the friends, the books and magazines that you can draw on as you go beyond The Winning Weigh. You now have the basic tools to be successful. Read and reread this book to help you digest all that it has to say. Then, go beyond this knowledge by adapting it to your unique goals and potential. Good luck, and remember that each moment is an opportunity to change. Each day is a new lifetime. Seize each moment, live fully every day, and your ultimate goal of a happy life will naturally follow.

Starting Right Now...

Start right now!

Summary of Step 7

1. Step 7 completes your new wellness role. Your daily review of your goals establishes the plans for this new you. Your daily visualization of your wellness image breathes life into this role. By filling out the Daily Food, Fiber, and Activity Journal, you see yourself acting out your new approach to living.

2. On a weekly basis your commitment to exercise will support and nurture your moment-to-moment commitments. Record your exercise sessions to discourage yourself from procrastinating.

3. People, the written word, pictures, and tapes can all help strengthen and support the growing, enhanced, new you.

4. Wellness is the active pursuit of mental, physical and spiritual health every day.

Appendix
The Winning Weigh Booster Plan

After a few months, you will probably find yourself beginning to waiver slightly from the wellness program you intended to follow. Use this Booster Plan to help yourself refocus on your health objectives. For three days, you will reaffirm your health goals while you are spring-cleaning your body and mind.

The three-day Booster Plan prescribes a variety of complex-carbohydrate foods to build up your tissue stores of anti-cancer nutrients. Your body will get a booster shot to assist in quenching, neutralizing, and detoxifying various free radicals and volatile environmental toxins. Think of it as building up your stock of ammunition in anticipation of an enemy attack.

We suggest that you use the Booster Plan four times a year, perhaps at the start of each new season. You should not use the Booster Plan for more than three consecutive days. ***It is not designed to be a long-term program,*** but rather to be a complement to the Winning Weigh program.

Prepare for the Booster Plan by reviewing your short-term goals. You want to involve both your mind and your body in this exercise. This would also be a good time to reread ***The Winning Weigh.*** As well as getting you back on track, a review of the book will give you the opportunity to remind yourself of facts you have forgotten and adopt ideas that may have seemed too drastic for you three months earlier. Rereading ***The Winning Weigh*** will help you develop strategies to cope with any new difficulties you are experiencing.

When you have your goals firmly in mind, commit yourself to the Booster Plan for three days.

The Booster Plan

Breakfast
- 1/2 lemon squeezed into a glass of water*
  (drink 15 minutes before eating)
- 8 - 10 oz. glass of pure carrot or papaya juice
- 3 - 4 oz. low-fat ricotta or cottage cheese, or
  8 oz. low-fat plain yogurt (1% M.F. or less)

Between Breakfast and Lunch
- 8 - 10 oz. of one of the following juices diluted with water*:
  - orange juice
  - grapefruit juice
  - carrot juice
  - pineapple juice

Lunch
- 2 cups Winning Weigh Vegetable Broth (see facing page)
- one serving of Winning Weigh Super Salad
  (see facing page)
- whole wheat roll
- 16 - 20 oz. water*

Between Lunch and Dinner
- one apple
- 16 - 20 oz. water*

Dinner
- 2 cups Winning Weigh Vegetable Broth
- 1/2 baked squash
- one serving of Bean Salad (see page 292)
- 1/2 cup brown rice (measure before cooking)
- 16 - 20 oz. of water*

One or Two Hours after Dinner
- 2 cups fruit salad, including any combination of the following: oranges, cantaloupe, honeydew, peaches, nectarines, apples, strawberries, mangoes, blueberries, watermelon
- 16 - 20 oz. of water*

* Do not drink tap water during this three-day period. Instead, drink distilled water, spring water, low-sodium mineral water, or low-sodium soda water.Drink as much water as you can, at least six glasses each day.

The Winning Weigh's Protective Nutrient Vegetable Broth
Makes enough for one person for one day.
7 carrots, 1 small bunch celery, 1/2 tomato, large handful fresh spinach, 1/3 bunch parsley, onion, okra, tomato, green pepper (you can decide how much you'd like of these vegetables), salt or garlic
- Finely chop all the vegetables.
- Place the carrots, celery, and tomato in two quarts (2 L) of hot water and boil for 15 minutes.
- Add the parsley and spinach. Boil for 10 more minutes.
- Place everything in a blender and purée until smooth and thick.

The Winning Weigh's Protective Nutrient Super Salad
Cook 1/2 cup of pasta per serving (measured before cooking). Refrigerate for at least three hours.
Toss together cauliflower, broccoli, green peppers, red peppers, tomatoes, carrots, celery, and cucumber in whatever proportions appeal to you.
Add the pasta and dress the salad with 2 tsp. olive oil and vinegar per serving.

The Winning Weigh's Protective Nutrient Bean Salad
Makes one serving.
> 1/4 cup chick-peas, cooked
> 1/4 cup red kidney beans, cooked
> 1 tsp olive oil and vinegar

- Toss the beans with the dressing.

Starting Now . . .

Follow the Winning Weigh Booster Plan every three months. Think of it as spring cleaning for your body. Try scheduling it along with a review of your short-term goals and a rereading of **The Winning Weigh.**

The Fiber Scoreboard

The following Fiber Scoreboard is based on the combined studies of Southgate et al, Anderson et al, Pope-Cordle and Katahn, Theander and Amon, the USDA Nutrient Data Research Group, and labelling information on brand-name foods. In order to keep the scoreboard simple and easy to use, we have rounded off some figures. You will find The Winning Weigh's Fiber Scoreboard a practical and reliable method of determining your overall fiber intake from day to day.

You should accumulate 8 to 15 fiber points per day to live up to the recommendations of the Cancer and Heart associations and other leading authorities.

For any food not listed here, divide the number of grams of fiber by three in order to determine the number of Winning Weigh fiber points.

The Fiber Scoreboard

Cereal Products	Portion Size	Calories	Fiber Points
Kellogg's All Bran	1/2 cup	90	3.5
Kellogg's Bran Buds	1/2 cup	90	3.5
Cooked buckwheat groats (kasha)	1 cup	160	3.0
Cooked bulgur	1 cup	160	3.0
Nabisco 100% Bran	1/2 cup	105	3.0
Cooked oatmeal	3/4 cup	212	2.5
Quaker Corn Bran	2/3 cup	115	2.0
Kellogg's Bran Flakes – plain	1 cup	90	1.5
– with raisins	1 cup	110	2.0
Most	1 cup	200	2.5
Kellogg's Bran Chex	2/3 cup	90	1.5
Fruitful Bran	3/4 cup	110	1.5
Shredded Wheat – large biscuit	1	74	0.75
– spoon size	1 cup	168	1.5
General Foods' Grape Nuts	1/4 cup	105	1.0
Health Valley Sprouts (7 with raisins)	1/4 cup	105	1.5
Kellogg's 40% Bran Flakes	3/4 cup	95	2.0
Quaker Oats – Life	2/3 cup	110	1.0
Kellogg's Nutri-Grain	2/3 cup	110	1.0
Kellogg's Nutri-Grain Wheat	3/4 cup	105	1.0
Post 40% Bran Flakes	2/3 cup	95	2.0
Quaker 100% Natural Cereal	1/4 cup	110	1.0
Kellogg's Special K	1 cup	105	0.25
Kellogg's Total	1 cup	115	1.0
Purina Wheat Chex	2/3 cup	105	1.0
Wheaties	1 cup	115	1.0
Kellogg's Corn Flakes	3/4 cup	70	1.0
Kellogg's Cracklin' Oat Bran	1/2 cup	110	1.0

Cereal Products	Portion Size	Calories	Fiber Points
Kellogg's Fruit N' Fiber	1/2 cup	90	1.0
Puffed Wheat	1 cup	43	1.0
Kellogg's Raisin Bran	1/2 cup	95	1.0
Cooked wheat	2/3 cup	101	0.75
Honey Nut Cheerios	3/4 cup	115	0.5
Honey Nut Crunch Raisin Bran	1/2 cup	95	0.5
Kellogg's Corn Pops	1 cup	105	0.25
Purina Corn Chex	1 cup	115	0.25
Cheerios	1/2 cup	60	0.25
Post Toasties Corn Flakes	1/2 cup	60	0.5
Hot Cereals			
Old Fashioned Quaker Oats	3/4 cup	110	1.0
Quick Quaker Oats	3/4 cup	110	1.0
Fruits			
Apple (raw)	1 med.	70	1.0
	1 large	80-100	1.5
Apple sauce	1/2 cup	115	0.5
Apricots (whole, raw)	1	17	0.5
Avocado	1 med.	306	1.0
Banana	1 med.	105	1.0
Blackberries	1/2 cup	27	1.5
Blueberries	1 cup	82	2.0
Boysenberries	1 cup	66	2.0
Cantaloupe	1 cup	57	0.5
Cherries	10	49	0.5
Cranberries (raw)	1/4 cup	12	0.5
Cranberry sauce	1/2 cup	246	1.0
Dates (pitted)	2	39	0.5

	Portion Size	Calories	Fiber Points
Figs (dried)	3	120	3.5
Figs (fresh)	1	30	0.5
Grapefruit (whole)	1	80	0.5
Grapes (white, red, or black)	15-20	70	0.5
Honeydew melon	3" slice	42	0.5
Kiwi	1 med.	46	0.5
Mango	1 med.	135	1.25
Nectarine	1 med.	67	1.0
Orange	1 large 1 small		
Papaya	1 med.	117	1.0
Passion fruit	1 med.	18	1.0
Peach – raw	1 med.	38	0.75
– canned in syrup	2 halves	70	0.5
Pear	1 med.	98	1.5
Persimmon	1 med.	32	1.0
Pineapple – raw	1/2 cup	41	0.5
– canned	1/2 cup	60-75	0.5
Plums	1 med.	36	0.5
Pomegranate	1 med.	104	0.75
Prunes (pitted)	3	122	0.75
Raisins	1 tbsp. 1/2 cup	29 192	0.5 1.25
Raspberries (raw, fresh, or frozen)	1/2 cup	20	1.5
Raspberry jam	1 tbsp.	75	0.5
Rhubarb (stewed)	1 cup	104	0.75
Strawberries (raw)	1 cup	45	1.0
Strawberry jam	1 tbsp.	90	0.5
Tangerine	1 med.	37	1.0
Watermelon	1 thick slice	68	0.5

	Portion Size	Calories	Fiber Points
Packaged/Prepared Fruits			
Birds Eye frozen strawberries (in syrup)	1/2 cup	160	0.5
Del Monte Bartlett pear halves	1/2 cup	80	0.75
Del Monte fruit cocktail	1/2 cup	80	0.25
Del Monte pineapple chunks (own juice)	1/2 cup	70	0.5
Del Monte sliced pineapple (own juice)	1/2 cup	70	0.5
Del Monte yellow cling peach halves	1/2 cup	50	1.0
Dale sliced pineapple	1/2 cup	95	0.5
Dale sliced pineapple (own juice)	1/2 cup	70	0.5
Libby's fruit cocktail	1/2 cup	85	0.5
Libby's Lite yellow cling peaches (packed in fruit juice)	1/2 cup	50	0.5
Sun Sweet whole prunes	5-6	120	3.0
Vegetables			
Artichoke – boiled	1 med.	53	1.0
– hearts	1/2 cup	37	0.75
Asparagus	1/2 cup	15	0.5
Avocado	1 med.	310	2.0
Bamboo shoots	1/2 cup	21	0.75
Beets	1/2 cup	33	1.0
Broccoli	1/2 cup	20	1.0
Broccoli spears	2	20	1.0
Brussels sprouts (cooked)	3/4 cup	36	1.0
Cabbage (raw or cooked)	1/2 cup	8	0.5
Carrots	1/4 cup	10	0.5

	Portion Size	Calories	Fiber Points
Carrot sticks	4-5	10	0.5
Carrots (cooked)	1/2 cup	20	0.5
Cauliflower (raw or cooked)	1 cup	16	1.0
Celery	1/4 cup	5	0.5
Celery stalks	1	8	0.5
Chinese-style vegetables	1/2 cup	79	1.0
Corn – popcorn	4 cups	90	2.0
– corn on the cob	1 med.	70	1.5
– cooked or canned	1/2 cup	64	1.5
Cucumber (raw)	1/2 med.	8	0.5
Eggplant	2 slices	42	1.0
Endive (raw)	20 leaves	10	0.5
Cooked greens: collards, beet greens, dandelion, kale, Swiss chard, turnip greens	1/2 cup	20	1.0
Lettuce (Boston, leaf, or Iceberg)	1 cup	10	0.5
Mushrooms	5 small	14	0.5
	10 small	28	1.0
Okra (raw, cooked, or frozen)	1/2 cup	13	0.5
Onion	1 med.	65	0.75
Parsley (chopped)	4 tbsp.	4	0.5
Parsnip (cooked)	1 large	76	1.0
Peas and carrots (frozen)	1/2 pkg.	40	2.0
Peppers	1/2 cup	13	0.5
Dried crushed peppers	1 tsp.	7	0.5
Potatoes	1 small	95	1.0
Radishes	3	5	0.25
Rhubarb (cooked)	1/2 cup	100	1.0
Rutabaga	1/2 cup	40	1.0
Sauerkraut (canned)	2/3 cup	15	1.0

	Portion Size	Calories	Fiber Points
Spinach – raw	1 cup	8	1.0
– cooked	1/2 cup	26	2.5
Summer squash (boiled)	1/2 cup	14	0.75
Winter squash (baked)	1/2 cup	63	1.0
Sweet potato (baked)	1 large	254	1.75
Tomatoes	1 small	22	0.5
	1/2 cup	22	0.5
Turnip – raw	1/4 cup	8	0.5
– cooked	1/2 cup	16	0.75
Watercress (raw)	1/2 cup	4	0.5
Yams (cooked or baked in skin)	1 med.	156	2.0
Zucchini (raw)	1/2 cup	11	0.75
Canned Vegetables, Peas, and Beans			
Del Monte cream style golden sweet corn	1/2 cup	80	1.0
Del Monte Early Garden spinach	1/2 cup	25	2.0
Del Monte Early Garden sweet peas	1/2 cup	60	2.0
Del Monte whole green beans	1/2 cup	20	1.0
Del Monte whole kernel Family Style corn	1/2 cup	70	1.0
Green Giant asparagus cuts	1/2 cup	20	1.0
Green Giant cream style corn	1/2 cup	100	1.0
Green Giant french style cut green beans	1/2 cup	18	1.0
Green Giant kitchen cut green beans	1/2 cup	20	1.0
Green Giant mushrooms	2 oz.	14	0.5
Green Giant sweet peas	1/2 cup	60	1.75
Green Giant whole kernel corn	1/2 cup	90	1.5

	Portion Size	Calories	Fiber Points
Le Sueur Early June peas (Pillsbury)	1/2 cup	60	2.0
Libby's Natural Pack mixed vegetables	1/2 cup	60	1.0
Veg-All (The Larsen Co.)	1/2 cup	35	1.0
Frozen Vegetables			
Birds Eye broccoli spears	1/2 cup	25	1.0
Birds Eye cooked winter squash	1/2 cup	45	1.0
Birds Eye cut green beans	1/2 cup	25	1.0
Birds Eye green peas	1/2 cup	80	2.0
Birds Eye Italian Style vegetables	1/2 cup	110	1.0
Birds Eye Japanese Style vegetables	1/2 cup	100	1.0
Birds Eye Little Ears of Corn	2 ears	130	1.5
Birds Eye San Francisco Style vegetables	1/2 cup	100	0.75
Birds Eye sweet corn	1/2 cup	80	1.75
Seabrook Farms baby Brussels sprouts	1/2 cup	35	1.0
Legumes (Peas and Beans)			
Black beans (cooked)	1/2 cup	100	3.0
Broad beans	3/4 cup	30	1.0
Northern navy beans	1 cup	160	5.0
Kidney beans	1/2 cup	150	3.0
Lima beans	1/2 cup	90	2.5
Pinto beans	1/2 cup	75	3.0
White beans – dried before cooking	1/2 cup	160	5.0
– dried, canned, cooked	1/2 cup	80	2.5
Bean sprouts (raw)	1/4 cup	7	1.0
Chick-peas (garbanzo beans) – canned or cooked	1/4 cup	205	2.0
Chestnuts	3 large	29	1.0

	Portion Size	Calories	Fiber Points
Green (snap) beans (fresh or frozen)	1/2 cup	10	0.75
Lentils	1/2 cup	100	1.0
Peas (green, fresh or frozen)	1/2 cup	60	3.0
Black-eyed peas (frozen or canned)	1/2 cup	74	2.5
Split peas (dried or cooked)	1/2 cup	63	2.0
Breads			
Bagel – plain	1	150	0.5
– whole wheat, pumpernickel	1	150	1.0
Boston brown bread	2 slices	100	1.0
Bread sticks	1	23	trace
Bulgur, dry	1 cup	548	4.5
Cornbread	1 piece	198	0.5
Cracked wheat bread	2 slices	120	1.0
Dark rye (whole grain) bread	2 slices	108	1.0
Dinner rolls	2	155	0.5
English muffins (whole wheat)	1	125	1.0
High-bran bread	2 slices	140	2.0
Pita – plain	1 large	240	0.5
– whole wheat	1 large	236	2.0
Pumpernickel	2 slices	116	1.0
Raisin bread	2 slices	140	0.75
Seven grain bread	2 slices	125	2.0
Sourdough bread	2 slices	136	0.5
White bread	2 slices	140	0.5
Whole wheat bread	2 slices	120	2.0
Whole wheat raisin bread	2 slices	140	2.0
Crackers			
Fiber Med biscuits	1	152	3.3
Graham crackers	3	53	0.75

	Portion Size	Calories	Fiber Points
Ry-Krisps	3	64	0.5
Triscuits	2	50	0.75
Wheat Thins	6	58	0.75
Premium Saltine crackers	10	120	0.5
UNEENA biscuits	6	130	0.5
Wasa Lite Rye Crispbread	3	90	1.0
Pasta			
Macaroni			
– whole wheat, uncooked	1/2 cup	200	2.0
Spaghetti			
– whole wheat (uncooked)	1/2 cup	200	1.5
– plain (uncooked)	1/2 cup	200	1.0
– with tomato sauce	1/2 cup	220	2.0
Spinach noodles (uncooked)	1/2 cup	200	2.0
Spinach lasagna	1 serving	215	1.0
Tortellini with tomato sauce	1 cup	317	0.5
Rice			
White (uncooked)	1/2 cup	79	0.75
Brown (uncooked)	1/2 cup	83	2.0
Instant rice	1 serving	79	0.25
Prepared Frozen Dinners			
(most are extremely high in salt)			
Armour Chicken Burgundy Classic Lite Dinner	11 1/4 oz.	240	2.0
Armour Chicken Fricassee Dinner Classic	11 3/4 oz.	330	2.0
Armour Seafood Natural Herbs Classic Lite Dinner	11 1/2 oz.	230	1.5
Armour Seafood Newburg Dinner Classic	10 1/2 oz.	270	1.0

	Portion Size	Calories	Fiber Points
Armour Sliced Beef with Broccoli Classic Lite	10 1/4 oz.	290	1.0
Norton Turkey Dinner	11 oz.	340	1.0
Swanson Hungry-Man Turkey Dinner	18 1/2 oz.	630	2.0
Swanson Macaroni and Cheese Dinner	12 1/4 oz.	380	2.0
Swanson Turkey Dinner	11 1/2 oz.	340	2.0
Stouffer's Glazed Chicken with Vegetable Rice Lean Cuisine	8 1/2 oz.	270	0.5
Stouffer's Spaghetti with Beef and Mushroom Sauce Lean Cuisine	11 1/2 oz.	280	0.5
Soups			
Campbell's Chunky Vegetable Soup	1 cup	104	1.0
Progresso Minestrone Soup	8 oz.	130	1.75
Progresso Green Split Pea Soup	1 cup	180	1.75
Potato soup	1 cup	178	2.75
Prepared Dinner			
Ratatouille	1/2 cup	87	0.5
Mexican Foods (low in fat, high in fiber)			
Bean burrito (without cheese)	1 large	284	2.0
Old El Paso Refried Beans	1 cup	200	4.0
Oriental Foods			
Chicken and vegetable stir fry	1 cup	142	1.0
Chop suey or chow mein	1 cup	?	0.75
Chun King Chicken Chow Mein Pouch	6 oz.	90	1.0
La Choy Fancy Chinese Mixed Vegetables (drained)	1/2 cup	12	1.0
La Choy Shrimp Chow Mein	3/4 cup	60	0.5
La Choy Sukiyaki	3/4 cup	70	1.0

The Wellness Planner

My Wellness Starting Point

Fill in the following chart, giving the objective information as well as your *feelings* about some aspects of your life.

Date:

Weight:

Measurements:
    Waist: Hips:
    Chest: Thighs:

Health problems:

Diseases that people in my family have suffered from:

Medical information (e.g., blood pressure, cholesterol count, etc.):

Energy level:

Amount and quality of sleep:

Fitness routine:

Complex Carbohydrates

On one side of the page, list all the protein and high-fat foods that you will start eliminating from your diet. On the other side, list all the health-promoting, high-fiber, cancer-combatting complex carbohydrate foods you are going to eat instead.

I Am Going to Eat Less of the Following Foods

I Am Going to Eat More of These Complex Carbohydrates

Fiber

The following foods are high in fiber. Check off the ones that you intend to eat more often. Add your own favorites to the list if they are not there now.

Cholesterol Crunchers

Apples	Potatoes
Pears	Plums
Oranges	Grapefruit
Berries	Carrots
Peaches	Peas
Beans	Oat bran
Oatmeal	Pumpernickel bread

Colon Cleaners

Whole grain bread	Wheat bran
Bran cereals	Rice bran
Brown rice	Puffed rice
Whole rice crackers	Corn bran
Corn	Popcorn
Cornmeal	Corn flakes
Peas	Beans

Fats

List all the high-fat foods that you eat now. Put an asterisk next to those that you eat often or that you think will be especially hard to give up. Try to think of a wellness-oriented food that you can substitute for each high-fat food, and list it in the right-hand column. (There are more ideas on substitutions in Step 3.)

High-Fat Foods I'll Avoid Starting Now   **Wellness Foods I'll Focus on Starting Now**

e.g., hamburgers   chicken breasts

Protein

List some ways you are going to prepare the following low-fat flesh protein and low-fat dairy protein foods. (You should try to make sure your meal plans are health-promoting.)

Chicken:

Turkey:

Fish:

Seafood:

Low-fat cheese:

Focusing on the Benefits

The following is a list of the benefits you can reap by living a wellness lifestyle. How do you feel about attaining these benefits? Some benefits will be more important to you than others. Take a few minutes to write down how you feel about each one. Rate each for importance, on a scale of one to five. This exercise will give you an idea of where to focus your energies.

1   Not important to me at all
2   I am a little concerned
3   Moderately important to me
4   I am quite concerned
5   Extremely important to me

Avoiding Cardiovascular Diseases

High blood pressure	1	2	3	4	5
High blood cholesterol	1	2	3	4	5
Strokes	1	2	3	4	5
Heart attack	1	2	3	4	5
Angina	1	2	3	4	5

Avoiding Lifestyle-Related Cancers

Lung cancer	1	2	3	4	5
Colon cancer	1	2	3	4	5
Stomach cancer	1	2	3	4	5
Ovarian cancer	1	2	3	4	5
Prostate cancer	1	2	3	4	5
Breast cancer	1	2	3	4	5
Uterine cancer	1	2	3	4	5
Skin cancer	1	2	3	4	5

Avoiding Other Health Problems

Osteoporosis	1	2	3	4	5
Mature-onset diabetes	1	2	3	4	5
Constipation	1	2	3	4	5
Excessive fatigue	1	2	3	4	5
Mild depression	1	2	3	4	5
Anxiety	1	2	3	4	5

Improving Physical Well-Being

Fitness level	1	2	3	4	5
Quality of sleep	1	2	3	4	5
Energy level	1	2	3	4	5
Physical appearance	1	2	3	4	5
Body shape	1	2	3	4	5
Weight loss	1	2	3	4	5
Weight gain	1	2	3	4	5
Athletic performance	1	2	3	4	5

Improving Psychological Well-Being

Self-confidence	1	2	3	4	5
Vitality	1	2	3	4	5
Concentration	1	2	3	4	5
Starting new activities	1	2	3	4	5
Meeting new people	1	2	3	4	5

Making the Program Work Every Day

List all the Recreational Foods and Hazardous Foods that you eat now. Beside each one, write a Winning Weigh substitution from the list of Wellness or Compromise Foods that you will start eating instead.

Recreational Foods   **Substitutions**

Hazardous Foods   **Substitutions**

Preparing Food on the Winning Weigh

Write down some preparation hints (from Step 3) that you are going to incorporate into your cooking style.

Your Mission Statement

A mission statement is a single sentence that describes your life as you want it to be. Writing a mission statement for yourself will help you focus your efforts. It may take you a few tries to capture your main goals in a single sentence, so make your first attempts on a scrap piece of paper. When you have created a sentence that really feels right for you, copy it onto this page. Reread it often, and rewrite it if you find that it no longer adequately provides you direction and a sense of purpose.

Your Roles

Describe what you are like during the Perfect Forever act.

Describe yourself during the Blissful Binge act.

My Sedentary Slob

Write a detailed description of your Sedentary Slob. Use your imagination – go wild! You can even draw a picture of it. How big is it? What does its face look like? What color is it? Does it have a shape? Does it have hands or feet? Is it wearing clothes? You can also write a few scenarios for your Sedentary Slob to participate in.

Your Sedentary Slob Activators

List your Sedentary Slob activators in each of the three categories given: situations, people, and feelings. Take your time and be as specific as possible. Add to the list whenever you discover more details about your Sedentary Slob activators.

Situations
(e.g., going on vacation)

Specific Examples
(I feel I can eat whatever I want because I'm on holiday.)

People
(e.g., my mother)

Specific Examples
(She constantly criticizes the way I dress.)

Feelings
(e.g., self-indulgence)

Specific Examples
(I feel stuck at home with my work and the kitchen's always nearby.)

Discovering Your Sedentary Slob Beliefs

The following open-ended sentences are designed to give you a further understanding of your Sedentary Slob and Self-Righteous Snob roles. Think of yourself as an explorer about to map out an uncharted land. Sit back and complete the following statements with the first words and phrases that come to mind. These are just a few ideas to help get you started. You can apply the same general principles to discover your other beliefs about wellness.

Fat people are . . .

Dieting is . . .

Healthy foods are . . .

Unhealthy foods are . . .

Exercise is . . .

Lazing around all day is . . .

Out-of-shape people are . . .

Fried foods are . . .

Vegetables are . . .

Aerobic exercise is . . .

Going for walks is . . .

Thinking Styles

The more you know about your thinking styles, the better you will be prepared to deal with your Sedentary Slob and Self-Righteous Snob. Begin to collect your automatic thoughts and write them down under the appropriate category.

1. Procrastinated Success

2. Feeling Forecasting

3. Disaster Thinking

4. Blaming Others

5. Blaming Yourself

6. Weak and Dizzy

7. Never, Ever Again

8. And They Lived Happily Ever After

9. Doing/Undoing

10. Eureka

Wellness Affirmations

Write down your wellness affirmations in the space below so that you can refer back to them as often as necessary (see page 214).

Your Wellness Image

Once you have finished developing your first Wellness Image, write it down so you can refer back to it. Re-record your Wellness Image as it changes. Sign and date each entry.

Visualizing Your High-Risk Situations

Look back at your list of Sedentary Slob activators. For each one, create a personalized, detailed plan for dealing with it successfully the next time it arises. Describe as many details as you can, including the setting and the time of day you are most likely to encounter the activator. Use these descriptions in your daily visualization sessions to learn to make health-promoting choices.

The Daily Food, Fiber, and Activity Journal

Date: _____

Food and Beverages	Fiber Points	Activity
Breakfast: CC = 1/2 cup All Bran cereral DP = 8 oz. of skim milk CC = 1 slice whole wheat toast with CC = whole fruit jam NCB = black coffee	3.5 1 0.5	*Type:* Power Walk *Distance:* 3 Miles *Duration:* 45 Minutes
Lunch: FP = 1 small tin water packed salmon CC = 1 bagel CC = fruit cup NCB = low salt soda water	 1 1	
Dinner: CC = 1 cup spaghetti with tomato sauce CC = 1 white roll CC = mixed salad with olive oil & vinegar NCB = diet drink	2 0.5 1	
(8 to 15) **Total Fiber Points**	10.5	

Read Your Goals ___ Visualize ___ Exercise ___
Fill Out Your Dietary Record ___

In The Moment Diary

Situation	Intensity Level	Technique	Outcome	Next Time I'll...
Wedding dessert table, wanted pastries	Overwhelming	Talking your way out–"Make my day"	Chose fruit	Do the same
Poker night– eating what they are serving	Insufficient	Thinking your way out	ate chips, dip, ice cream etc. (unsuccessful outcome)	(i) Perform stepping back & breathing technique (ii) Use seeing your way out

The Daily Food, Fiber, and Activity Journal

Date: _____

Food and Beverages	Fiber Points	Activity
		Type: *Distance:* *Duration:*
(8 to 15) **Total Fiber Points**		

Read Goals ___ **Visualize** ___ **Exercise** ___
Fill Out Dietary Record ___

In The Moment Diary

Situation	Intensity Level	Technique	Outcome	Next Time I'll...

Weekly Body Shape Summary

Date (Week ending): _____

Exercise Summary:

No. of Aerobic Workouts _____

Total Distance (jogged/walked) _____

No. of Recreational Sports _____

Weight _____ lbs. (kg)

Waist _____ in. (cm)

Hips _____ in. (cm)

Upper Thigh _____ in. (cm)

Chest (M) _____ in. (cm)

Bicep _____ in. (cm)

Calf _____ in. (cm)

Weekly Body Shape Summary

Date (Week ending): _____

Exercise Summary:

No. of Aerobic Workouts　　　　　_____

Total Distance (jogged/walked)　　_____

No. of Recreational Sports　　　　_____

Weight	_____	lbs. (kg)
Waist	_____	in. (cm)
Hips	_____	in. (cm)
Upper Thigh	_____	in. (cm)
Chest (M)	_____	in. (cm)
Bicep	_____	in. (cm)
Calf	_____	in. (cm)

NOTES

NOTES

NOTES